"We know that exercise is key for goldeners, but in *Dynamic Aging*, Bowman and her impressive coauthors go one step further. They show how movement, not just exercise, is key to living dynamically, well into your seventh, eighth, and ninth decades. Essential reading for both goldeners and the fitness professionals that work with them."

— Sandy Todd Webster, Editor in Chief, *IDEA Fitness Journal*

"Aging is not about age—poor movement habits age and derail us. Our vitality is never wholly lost and can be regained by coaching joints and muscles toward their ability to function optimally."

—Michele Olson, PhD, The Exercise Doctor, Professor of Exercise Physiology and a Fellow of the ACSM

"Nothing makes me happier than getting people walking. With *Dynamic Aging*, more people will be able to walk, walk farther, and enjoy it even more. This is sure to help many, many people of all ages."

—Leslie Sansone, creator of the Walk at Home programs

"Yes! *Dynamic Aging* makes it clear it's never too late to start moving BETTER. This easy-to-understand book is sure to benefit many who may have thought their days of moving with ease have passed."

—Tamilee Webb, MA, star of BUNS OF STEEL™ and author of *The Original Rubber Band Workout*

"*Dynamic Aging* shifts the conversation from exercising to moving. Her goldener coauthors are living proof this works, no matter when one starts. Aging is not a choice. How we age is!"

—Kathy Smith, New York Times bestselling author, recipient of IDEA lifetime achievement award

ALSO BY KATY BOWMAN

Movement Matters

Simple Steps to Foot Pain Relief

Diastasis Recti

Don't Just Sit There

Whole Body Barefoot

Move Your DNA

Alignment Matters

DYNAMIC AGING

AGING

Simple Exercises for Whole-Body Mobility

By Katy Bowman

With Joan Virginia Allen, Shelah M. Wilgus,
Lora Woods, and Joyce Faber

PROPRIOMETRICS
PRESS

Printed in the United States of America.
Fourth Printing, 2017
ISBN paperback: 978-1-943370-11-5
Library of Congress Control Number: 2016962297
Propriometrics Press: propriometricspress.com
    Cover and Interior Design: Zsofi Koller, zsofikoller.com
    Illustrations: Jillian Nichol
    Front Cover Photo: John Eder Photography
    Back Cover Photo: Michael Curran
    Author Photos, Goldeners: Cecilia Ortiz
    Author Photo, Katy Bowman: J. Jurgensen Photography
    Diagram on pg. 120: Teguh Mujiono/Shutterstock
    Interior Image Treatment: Shelah M. Wilgus

The information in this book should not be used for diagnosis or treatment, or as a substitute
for professional medical care. Please consult with your healthcare provider prior to attempting any
treatment on yourself or another individual.

    Publisher's Cataloging-In-Publication Data
    (Prepared by The Donohue Group, Inc.)

    Names: Bowman, Katy. | Allen, Joan Virginia.
    Title: Dynamic aging : simple exercises for whole-body mobility / by Katy Bowman ; with
Joan Virginia Allen [and 3 others].
    Description: [Sequim, Washington] : Propriometrics Press, 2017. | Includes bibliographical
references and index.
    Identifiers: ISBN 978-1-943370-11-5 | ISBN 978-1-943370-12-2 (ebook)
    Subjects: LCSH: Exercise therapy for older people. | Older people--Orientation and mobility.
| Human locomotion. | Movement education. | Equilibrium (Physiology)
    Classification: LCC RC953.8.E93 B69 2016 (print) | LCC RC953.8.E93 (ebook) | DDC
613.7/10846--dc23

To Katy Bowman, whose paradigm of whole-body movement is a gift that opens the door to healing the cause of pain.

—J. F.

To my husband and soulmate, Willis. I love the adventure of life with you.

—J. V. A.

To Shelah, Joyce, Lora, and Joan, with my love and admiration.

—K. B.

To Gail Dennison, who sweetly yet consistently recommended that I try Katy Bowman's approach to joint care before resigning myself to surgery.

—L. W.

To Thea, who first found Katy, and Tessa, who gets me out walking.

—S. W.

TABLE OF CONTENTS

INTRODUCTIONS

When I was a kid, my mother observed that I "always insisted on learning the hard way," meaning that I wouldn't let myself benefit from the wisdom of others, and needed, instead, to experience lessons for myself. Fortunately, I've grown out of this trait in many respects. Now when I meet people who have had the experience of walking down a path I am currently on, I value their insight. And what I've learned from the people around me who've lived much longer than I have is that I need to take good care of my body, because if I don't, I'll miss being able to move how I want to.

I have had my body for only forty-one years, but over the last twenty-two, I've had the pleasure of working one-on-one with over a thousand bodies, most of them older than mine. And if there is one message I've received loud and clear, it's that those coming to me for corrective exercise and alignment work in their sixties and seventies wish they had had access to this material in their twenties. From these people, I've learned to value future physical function *now*. That's why I've chosen to write this book.

I teach people new ways to move their bodies. And I've had the good fortune of working with a large group of people over a long period of time. This means I have been exposed to a lot of data—about what people have done in the past, which hobbies and injuries they have, and where they are today.

I've worked with groups of competitive athletes, young children, pregnant mamas, post-natal mamas, and breast cancer survivors. I've led courses for those with cardiovascular disease, bad backs, and pelvic floor disorders, and thousands of people suffering with foot pain. I've gathered the information on what thousands of people have done in their past, and as a result, I've become familiar with the average movement history of today's seventy- and eighty-year-olds in my culture.

This book includes the stories of four of my clients: an attorney, a dance-movement therapist and RN, a teacher and social worker, and a sassy, kick-ass graphic artist (she's done most of the graphics in this book) who travels to far away countries. These women began working with me in their late sixties and early seventies and were part of a large group that started taking classes in my new-at-the-time exercise facility around a decade ago. They were the four who continued to show up, sometimes two hours a day Monday through Friday, for years, eventually studying to become movement teachers themselves.

Now, in their mid- to late seventies at time of writing (with one turning eighty just as this book is being published), they are some of the few of their own peer group who haven't made a transition into senior living centers. They look younger now than they did years ago. They move "younger" than they did years ago. I regularly tell people this is possible—that they can look, move, and feel younger through smart movement and regular training—but I'm forty-one years old. Who's going to believe me when I say that starting at sixty or even seventy isn't too late and that tremendous improvement is possible? And so I thought I would ask Joan, Lora, Joyce, and Shelah to share with you their own insights about how a goldener can turn back the clock. You'll see their commentary throughout the book, the perspectives of four strong, dedicated, powerful women well into their seventies who are active and thriving.

But what is a goldener? When these women came to me with the idea for this book, they were clear: *We don't want "old" in the title. Or "senior." Or "geriatric," for that matter. How about an all-new, beautiful term that describes how we feel about this stage of our lives, the golden age? How about "goldener"?* I agree wholeheartedly with their thoughtful word choices, and science seems to as well.

Exercise has powerful capabilities to improve health, but so do words. During a game of charades, have you ever mimed a senior, shuffling at a snail's pace, stooped over, one hand on the low back and the other on an imaginary cane? As biological beings, our behavioral patterns are shaped by what we see—how our own parents move, how our peers move. Even how cultural norms are portrayed on TV can shape our reality. The question is, how do other people move, and how do preconceived notions of the way the "over sixties" move affect how we move once we, ourselves, are older?

In a study created to measure the impact of positive or negative stereotype reinforcement, researchers found that walking speed and time spent in the balance phase of walking increased after only thirty minutes of intervention (Hausdorff, Levy, and Wei 1999). Did the researchers hand out a magical exercise or stretch? Nope. During a thirty-minute video game, subliminal terms were flashed on the screen: *senile, dependent, diseased* for one group and *wise, astute, accomplished* for the other. With absolutely no exercise intervention, the positively reinforced group was able to make gait and walking speed improvements more commonly found after weeks or even months of exercise training. So here's the takeaway message for everyone: Words can be profound, so practice positive speak about yourself and those around you. And here's the takeaway message for exercisers: The way you're moving (or not) right now could be influenced by things other than your physiology.

There are many headlines, some of them about research, announcing the norms of the human experience. However, using age as a variable in research can be problematic as it's hard to separate age from length of habit. There is a difference between the statements "Older adults are more prone to bunions" and "Older adults who've been wearing too-tight shoes for longer are more prone to bunions." Age is typically selected as a research variable because it is objective and easier to quantify than your behavior over time. You can tell me with great accuracy how old you are, but it's less likely you could tell me with great accuracy just how many hours you've spent with your toes crammed together in your shoes. And so, it is often through language in general and language used in research that we perpetuate the idea that bodies start falling apart simply because they've reached a certain age. Of course, all cells will eventually cease to replace themselves, but what's important here is not the inevitability of decline, but that we're able to see the difference between natural decline and the loss of function we're experiencing simply due to weaknesses created by poor movement habits.

And here's something else to consider: There seems to be a culture-wide decrease in strength that's not related to age, but to a lifestyle that requires very little movement. A study comparing the grip strength of millennials (those born between approximately 1980 and 2000) in 2015 to the grip strength of this same age group in 1985, for example, shows people's grips are significantly weaker today than they used to be (Fain and Weatherford 2016). Kids today (I never thought I'd type *those* words) move less than I did as a kid, and according to my grandparents, I moved less throughout my childhood than they did throughout theirs. Given the human timeline, i.e., the recent introduction of technology and the relatively recent Industrial Revolution, I'll suggest that with each generation comes less movement. This is actually good news, as it means our perception of the general decline in body weakness over time could very well be coming from the fact that we've really just been extremely sedentary the bulk of our lives. We're mostly *under-moved*, and not at all *too old*.

Dynamic Aging is a guide to get you moving more and moving more of you. This isn't a book that suggests, "Hey, you should start walking!" Instead, it helps you see which parts of your body you can start moving a tiny bit here and there so you feel like going out to take a walk. This guide contains exercises designed to improve your movement habits through simple postural adjustments and exercises designed to challenge your body, gently, in a way that you probably stopped doing a long time ago without realizing it. As you slowly introduce more movement into your life, it's likely you'll see an improvement in those movement declines that you had associated with age but that were actually a product of your long-term movement patterns.

This is a guide facilitated by four of the most amazing,

dynamic goldeners I know, who began just as you are about to now (with their feet). I hope you will gain as much from reading their experiences as I have from participating in them.

MEET THE GOLDENERS:

Joan

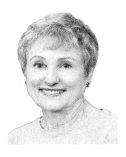

At the age of seventy-one, after a long career as an attorney, I was referred to Katy Bowman for exercises to help with my pelvic prolapse, chronic constipation, and foot problems. I met with her for a whole-body evaluation and began the movement practice that day which would change my life. I am now seventy-eight years of age. My chronic constipation completely disappeared three years into my movement practice. I walk daily and am able to continue to pursue my passion for hiking (three to ten miles), now in FiveFinger and zero-drop shoes, on the mountainous terrain of the trails on our ranch, on the sandy beaches of our nearby coast, and in our quest to hike all of the national parks (thirty-two to date, with the latest six hiked last summer in my seventy-ninth year). I can walk barefoot without discomfort. I climb and hang from trees in our forest—something I would never have thought of doing but for Katy's example and instruction. At seventy, I was scheduled for major surgery to address my pelvic organ prolapse. The surgery has not yet been necessary. My balance is the best it has ever been—about two years ago I walked barefoot across a log six feet above a rushing river, something I never thought I'd be able to do, and certainly not for the first time at age seventy-seven. That same year (2015), Joyce (then seventy-eight) and I walked the sands of the Dungeness Spit in Washington for a total of eleven miles to see the lighthouse. And my overall body strength has improved significantly.

Changing how I move has changed my life, and I now work as a movement teacher, sharing what I've learned with others.

Joyce

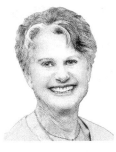

I sustained painful knee injuries twenty-nine years ago. I had completed my teaching career of twenty years and was in the process of getting my master's degree in social work when I injured the meniscus of my right knee doing yoga practice at home without the proper warm-up needed because of a studying, sitting, listening overload. The injuries I sustained—a meniscus torn in one knee and the other damaged shortly after from compensating stresses—are common. For years I sought relief from the pain and restricted mobility with a variety of palliative measures: limited walking, Tai Chi, gentle yoga stretching, daily pain pills, weekly chiropractic treatments, and massage therapy. Yet other than surgery—a choice I was unwilling to make due to the risk of complications and limited chance for sustained improvement—there appeared to be no path for healing and wellness. That all changed for me when

I was sixty-nine, and my chiropractor told me she would not continue to treat me unless I learned how to strengthen my muscles to keep the bones adjusted between our appointments. I did not want to lose my chiropractor, so when a friend told me about Katy Bowman's movement classes, I went. Almost immediately I began to understand my body from a biomechanical point of view. I learned that injuries, pain, and inflammation are our bodies' warning flags: we shouldn't ignore them or power through them, but rather teach ourselves to heal using them as our guides. This whole-body model of wellness has taught me that our health is influenced more by our habits—the way we use, load, and live in our body—than by our age. Today at age seventy-nine (I'll be eighty when this book is printed), without having had any surgery, I have regained my ability to walk without pain or impairment and to live with wellness in my body, mind, and spirit. Whole-body movement has made this possible in my life and I feel strong and capable walking the path to healing and wellness.

Lora

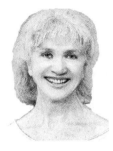

At sixty-eight, I was scheduled for the first of at least two surgeries that would have left me with a complete knee replacement. Through my work as an RN and dance-movement therapist, I thought I knew and had experienced all the self-help modalities and was resigned to "the knife." A friend talked me into trying Katy's exercise program. Although convinced that it was another incomplete answer, I decided I should try everything. And her program turned out to be just that: everything. I had endured restless leg syndrome since my teens (before it had a name). For six decades I lost an average of one night's sleep every two weeks to nerve pain originating in my sacrum. After doing some of her exercises for two weeks, I began noticing that I wasn't even getting twinges of my usual "restless leg." That was an amazing finding for me, as I'd thought it was a familial malady. This success empowered me to cancel knee surgery and more frequently try gentle knee-stretching exercises for my frozen knee. Currently, at seventy-five, I can walk up to six miles on any terrain, and walk to all my in-town errands and appointments on my original biological equipment.

More important to me even than that was my ability to pack into the Sierra Mountains. Last year, I was able to join my sons and some grandkids on a one-week, lake-to-lake adventure. I carried one-fifth of my weight in supplies over beautiful but sometimes rugged and steep terrain. I started out early each day and was the last to arrive at the next camp, but I still feel both lucky and triumphant. Incorporating the principles in this book into my daily activities has created opportunities to change life-long conditions I thought were "just me." My biggest reward, however, is the excitement of students who, like me, are finding that aging isn't bad after all—aging is an opportunity to move, play, and expand into new areas.

Shelah

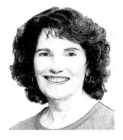

I started classes with Katy at age sixty-six, when I retired from my job as a graphic designer (sitting at a computer a lot). I'm a life-long exerciser, but I was so impressed with the logic of the scientific theory of her program, I decided to do more than the exercises—I decided to take her teacher training program.

I'm a work in progress and a product of my long-term habits. While preparing for a trip just before my seventy-fifth birthday, I reached into my closet trying to find a garment and twisted too far (not a Katy-recommended movement, for sure), and the resulting back pain made it obvious something was very wrong. Because I wanted to go on my trip, I treated the pain aggressively (bad move) and finally went to my family doctor. An MRI showed serious scoliosis in my back accompanied by painful shearing of lumbar vertebrae.

After a very long month of doctor-prescribed inactivity except five- to ten-minute walks on level ground, I was well enough to start the basic exercises you'll be learning in this book. Today at seventy-eight I can walk three to four miles daily in relative comfort. Healing at this stage of my life often takes a long time and, yes, it has tried my patience. Using the principles and exercises outlined here, my back is healing and I am slowly regaining my active lifestyle. Moving better doesn't automatically mean you don't get injured, but it makes you more resilient if you do. Katy's teaching has given me the knowledge and tools to know what movements I can do, like hanging and core strengthening, and which movements I must be very careful doing—like twisting.

Who Can Use this Book?

A book on dynamic aging is really for anyone, at any age. Truly, exercise programs should be geared to strength and skill levels rather than to any particular age, which can have little relevance to strength and skill levels, as you're about to find out. And so, this book could be easily utilized by anyone wanting to be more dynamic but feeling like they're starting from a place of little balance and strength.

Note From the Goldeners

This book is for readers of any age. Attaining and maintaining mobility, strength, and balance is a lifetime task. When we were young, we learned to balance, optimize our stability, stay on our feet for extended periods of time, and walk upright with confidence. Then, our lives took us in a more sedentary direction until, lo and behold, we found that easy movement had been lost somewhere along the way. We have learned so many exercises through our training with Katy, but the exercises in this book are those that we feel have been key to regaining and maintaining the balance and mobility lost to us through years of neglect.

Katy will be giving the more technical information and guidelines throughout this book, but this is what we septuagenarians have found helpful to keep in mind:

- Work to incorporate the basic alignment points and movements into your daily routine.
- Treat your body with appreciation and respect.
- Approach exercise with mindfulness, not force.
- Remember even small changes add up to larger functional improvements.

One job of your muscles is to stabilize your joints to allow full function of your entire musculoskeletal system. The exercises in this book are designed to mobilize and strengthen neglected muscles for the purpose of improving your head-to-toe alignment and day-to-day function.

SAFETY FIRST. It is always important to check with your doctor or physical therapist before beginning any exercise program, especially if you have "replacement" parts, including but not limited to hip replacements or knee replacements.

DISTINGUISH BETWEEN PAIN AND NEW SENSATIONS. If you experience pain while doing an exercise, try other options or modifications offered or come back in a few days, and try it again. You are the boss of you! Take responsibility for your own safety and well-being.

CRAMPING may occur when muscles are being stretched or used in different ways. If you experience cramping during an exercise, you may STOP doing the exercise and allow the muscles to relax before doing it again.

SORENESS after exercise may occur as a result of using muscles (and joints, bones, and fascia) in a new way and/or overusing your tissue (going too far too fast). Be gentle with yourself as you try these exercises. Go slowly, focus on what you are doing, and be mindful of what your body is experiencing. Adjust accordingly.

SAFETY TIP: For added stability while doing any standing evaluation or exercise, **we recommend you start by holding on to or leaning against a secure surface such as a counter, the back of a sofa, a wall, or a closed door to prevent falling**. While the overall goal is to do these exercises without support, safety and prudence should always be primary concerns.

SUGGESTED EQUIPMENT

- Thick and heavy book or yoga block

- Chair with straight back and level seat

- Rolled up towel or half foam roller (pictured below)

- Tennis ball

- Full-length mirror (very useful but not mandatory)

- Mat (optional)

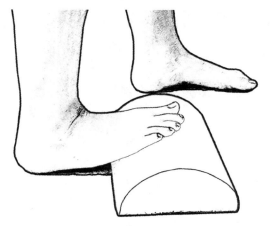

HALF FOAM ROLLER

CHAPTER 1
YOUR FEET ARE YOUR FOUNDATION

I love feet. In fact, I've written two whole books about them (*Simple Steps to Foot Pain Relief* and *Whole Body Barefoot*). You should love your feet too. Not only are they amazingly complex—they each have thirty-three joints and over a hundred muscles, tendons, and ligaments—but they also serve as the foundation to almost every day-to-day task you perform. This is why stiff, painful, under-moved feet are the first body part you should start moving better if you're finding your other parts—like knees and hips—difficult to move.

Even though most of what we do with our bodies—get up out of a chair, take a walk through the park, drive a car—requires we use our feet to a certain degree, we never really use the sophisticated machinery of our feet to their full potential. Instead, we use all of the many parts that make up our feet as one clump—one clump living inside of a shoe.

Chances are that you (like me until a few years ago, and probably also like almost everyone else you know) have spent the bulk of your life wearing "good" shoes. Stiff shoes. Supportive shoes. Shoes with elevated heels and limited space to stretch your toes. Shoes that, over decades, have sort of "casted" the muscles in your feet. This, combined with our excessive sitting and lack of walking on natural terrain (and many other habits we have), can lead to foot ailments such as bunions, hammertoes, bone spurs, plantar fasciitis, osteoarthritis, and neuropathy. If you don't move all of the joints and muscles in your feet, then your circulation decreases, which has big implications for your ability to heal from injuries, especially important to those dealing with diabetes. Our immobilized feet can also lead to ailments that don't seem immediately foot related—knee, hip, lower-back, and even neck pain can all be connected to your foot health.

Perhaps you've experienced so much pain that you've been prescribed special shoes or splints or orthotics; maybe you even have to limit your walking because of pain you've experienced.

But here's the good news: It's much more likely that your feet feel weak and stiff because you've spent a lifetime not using the muscles within them than it is your feet are weak and stiff solely due to their age.

Joan Says

I was always a barefoot girl. When I got into my forties, I began to notice pain in the balls of my feet when walking on a hard surface like a hardwood, tile, or concrete floor. Then I began noticing I could not walk barefoot at the beach without the balls of my feet hurting. I had never worn really high heels—nothing more than two inches. I was surprised and dismayed.

(sidebar cont'd next page)

(sidebar cont'd from previous page)

I was prescribed orthotics for my dressy work shoes AND for my sporty tennis shoes. I had to wear them in just about every shoe I owned. However, there didn't seem to be orthotics for heels. This created even more discomfort, because all my weight was being shoved down on the balls of my feet. I experienced pain when walking and standing and I got backaches. Whenever I could, I would slip off my shoes at work while sitting at my desk. And I wanted to sit a lot more of the time.

When I "retired" (left my lawyering days), I did a lot more Olympic-style race-walking and was paying well over $100 a pair for walking shoes that were engineered with air or other devices supposedly to protect my feet from feeling any pain. However, training for half marathons was not possible without orthotics. I finally resigned myself to the fact that I would wear orthotics for the rest of my life because I knew I wasn't getting any younger. And we all know it's all downhill physically as you get older (or so I had heard).

When I met with Katy for my first movement session, she explained the importance of getting my weight off the front of my feet and back onto my heels. For me this was a HUGE challenge because for nearly seventy years I had been standing with my pelvis forward, knees slightly bent, and weight on the balls of my feet. (It was as if I had a magnet in my belly that was constantly being

(sidebar cont'd next page)

pulled toward my kitchen counter when I was washing dishes or preparing food.) She suggested I try reducing the height of my heel, cautioning me to start out wearing flat shoes for only a short time at first to allow my feet and body to adjust to having my weight more on the rear of my foot. But I couldn't get the lower shoes to fit properly with my orthotics. She suggested I try my new shoes, along with my new exercises and foot mobility, without my orthotics. I was apprehensive but figured it would be self-limiting—if it hurt too much, I could just go back to my old shoes and orthotics.

Here we are, eight years later, and I've never gone back. Not only have I found it unnecessary to use my old whole-foot orthotics, I can again walk barefoot on the beach and for limited periods on the tile surfaces at home. Unfortunately, I have discovered the fat pads of the bottoms of my feet have either moved or disappeared, leaving my bones without cushions, so in my zero-drop and "barefoot" FiveFinger shoes, I now use a small, soft metatarsal pad and thin, flat liner pad cut just behind my toes to pad just under the soles of my feet. With this arrangement I hike three to five miles regularly on dirt trails, and do longer hikes in the nearby mountains and in the national parks. So not only has the condition of my feet improved, I am now doing something I never did before—using minimal shoes to improve my overall whole-body conditioning.

The following exercises are truly foundational in that they are designed to strengthen and mobilize the feet to improve their function and how they feel, but also in that larger movements

The Immobility Cycle

The longer we've been inactive, the less all our parts move, and the more we start doing things in our life that repeat the cycle. For example, sitting for long portions of each day for school and then work may have left the muscles in your legs weak, the joints in your knees and hips tight. When putting on a shoe every morning becomes a challenge—which is really another way of saying that moving in a particular way has become a challenge—we start opting for shoes that are easier to put on.

Shoes that require less hip and knee use are typically slip-ons, shoes that you can just poke your feet into. But here's the thing: Slip-on shoes could just as easily be called slip-OFF shoes, which is why, when you wear them, you have to clench your toes and stiffen the muscles in your feet and ankles just to keep them on. Stiff feet are weak feet—feet that aren't able to spread out into a wider, more stable base while you're walking and can't sense your environment and respond quickly.

While slippers and slide-on shoes are certainly a convenient way to address one consequence of stiff hips (i.e., difficulty putting on shoes), a "big picture" approach would be to work toward better hip mobility so that you don't end up adding "tight feet" and "decreased balance" to what started as just a hip issue (see page 132 for an exercise to address this).

and skills, like balance and walking, depend on well-functioning feet. We're used to approaching our health in segments. Foot exercises are for the feet, hip stretches benefit the hips, and balance exercises are to improve balance. While this is true, exercises for the feet can also benefit the hips and balance. The effects of movement are holistic in nature, so if you're thinking "my feet are fine, I want to jump to balance challenges," know that each exercise in this book directly impacts all other movements you'd like your body to be able to do, and starting with the feet can make a huge impact because, as I've already mentioned, most other things you do with your body begin at the feet.

Case in point, the first exercise for your feet isn't even a movement of the feet themselves: it's a movement of your hips.

WEAR YOUR HIPS OVER YOUR HEELS

Most of us have been wearing shoes with a heel. It doesn't matter if it's one inch or three, conventional shoes all come with raised heels and that has forced many of us to shift our pelves forward to balance out the downhill slope we've strapped to our feet. Line your hips up over your ankles.

BEFORE

AFTER

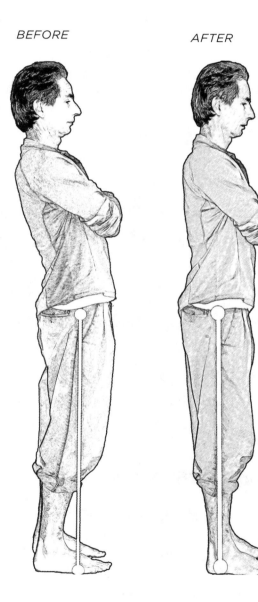

TOP OF THE FOOT STRETCH

The Top of the Foot Stretch stretches the muscles of your toes, feet, and ankles all at once, and targets any muscle clumps that might have developed due to too-tight shoes or postural habits. This stretch is key to improving toe, foot, and ankle mobility.

Begin by sitting near the front edge of a chair, feet flat on the floor. Reach back with one foot, tucking the toes under. Keep your heel centered; don't let your ankle flop to either side. Don't force the top of the foot to the floor in any way; allow your foot to lower as your tissues allow.

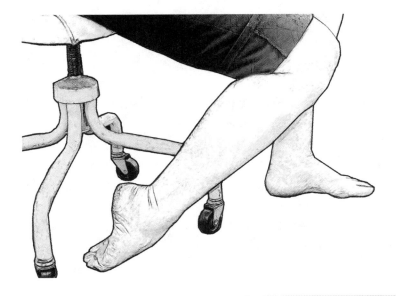

Once you can do this stretch with ease, it's time to try it standing up. Holding on to a wall or chair, reach your right foot behind you with the toes under, top of the foot stretching toward the floor. It's common at first to bend your torso slightly forward or shift your hips out in front to reduce the load to the feet. Notice these and try to bring your chest and hips back so they stack over your non-stretching foot. To make the foot stretch less you can always shorten the distance you've reached the leg back or return to the chair to lessen the load.

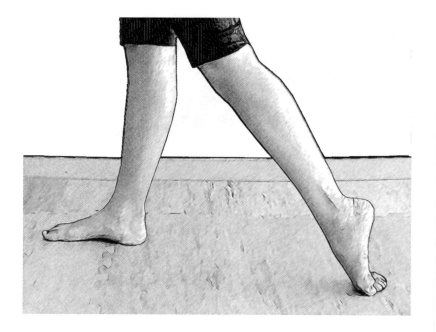

BOTTOM OF THE FOOT STRETCH

Walking on lumpy, bumpy terrain is something that, at a certain point, we start to avoid. Whether we're worried about falling or simply getting our shoes dirty, we tend to opt for flat and level paths for most of the walking we do. While I myself enjoy a smooth ride, the fact of the matter is we have thirty-three joints in each foot and between most of these are a lot of muscles that only get used when these joints change position.

Tip from the Goldeners

Important: Go slowly—you might not have moved these parts of your body in a long, long time. Find a "good" stretch in your foot and avoid taking the stretch to a place where you say, "ouch!" Stay present with what is happening in your body (i.e., don't do these while you're watching television), keeping your mind focused and able to monitor the feedback from this exercise. If your foot or calf muscles cramp, take your leg out of the stretch to relieve it, then return to the stretch as you can. Remember, many of us have not used these muscles for a long time, so expect some resistance. It is normal to experience cramping as these exercises are waking up long-underused muscles.

On Knees and Replacements

There are many types of joint replacements, each type having its own limits. Certain exercises can torque a joint more than others: we'll note these in bold so you can make sure to reduce your range of motion initially, move more slowly through these exercises, or discuss them directly with your orthopedic surgeon or physical therapist, who should be able to tell you the replacement type and movement limitations. For example, crossing one ankle over the other knee in a seated position as in the Toe Spreading exercise on page 38 could put certain types of hip replacements in a more vulnerable position. While waiting to discuss with your healthcare team, use the passive toe-spreading devices described on page 37 instead, which will keep you improving the mobility of this area until you determine if this exercise is a good fit for you. Look for bolded suggestions for those with joint replacements to steer you to alternate exercises.

It's easy to work your arm muscles by picking things up and setting them down, which in turn flexes and extends the elbow joint, but how do you bend the joints in the feet? It turns out that lumps and bumps on the ground do more than get in our way—they're how the smaller muscles in our feet get their exercise!

At this point, it's not necessary to strip off your shoes and go hike through a lumpy-bumpy meadow. Instead, you can more safely introduce low and controlled loads to your feet with a tennis or similarly sized squishy ball.

Start by sitting or standing and holding on to a secure surface (you choose which suits you best), and place the ball beneath one foot. Slowly load your weight onto the ball, moving your foot forward and back and side to side to apply pressure to individual joints within the foot.

Think of your foot as a floor you must vacuum. When it's your turn to vacuum, you don't just go around the edges, right? We don't vacuum along a single line down the middle of the floor—we vacuum all of it. Apply this diligence to your foot massage, moving tiny distances at a time, to leave no foot joint under-moved.

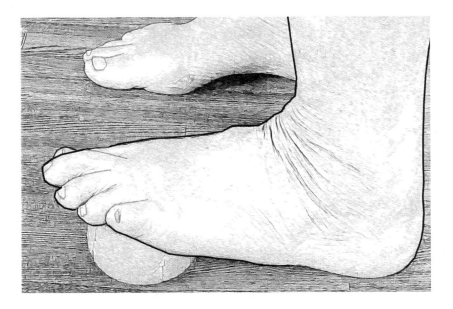

Work the entire sole of the foot with the ball, applying more or less pressure as needed. Standing places more weight (i.e., provides more foot-joint movement) than sitting, as does shifting more of your weight to the foot that's on the ball. Smaller and harder balls will create greater pressure (i.e., provide more movement) than larger, softer ones, so play around with different sizes and firmnesses, as each will mobilize the joints differently.

NOTE: Keep all of your balls and other exercise equipment in a basket, which will keep things from rolling underfoot when you're not expecting it!

STRETCH YOUR TOES FOR A WIDER BASE

The larger your base of support, the more balanced you'll be. This is often why we start turning our feet out as we walk—it provides us with a little more security in the moment, even though it can reduce ankle mobility in the long term. Chances are, right there in your shoes, are feet that are too narrow for your body. Not narrow by birth, but narrowed by too-tight shoes that have, over decades, squeezed your toes together. If you're experiencing issues with balance, take a look at your feet. Are they as wide, mobile, and strong as they could be?

To develop a wider base of support, you need to be able to spread your toes so that your entire foot covers more area. I know that narrow feet are often coveted for their appearance, but the fact of the matter is we don't want our balance to be dainty. We want to feel stable as we move from point A to point B, and this depends heavily on the shape and function of our feet.

TOE SPREADING

To see how quickly you can improve the function of your feet, begin with a self-assessment. You know how you can spread your fingers away from each other? You should be able to do that with your toes as well. To check your current ability, stand up unshod and see if you can move your toes away from each other. How'd you do?

It could be that although you're sending the "spread" signal to your feet, tissues there are too stiff to execute your command. Help out stiff toe-spreading muscles by giving them a hand. Literally. Sitting down, cross your right ankle over your left knee and hold the right foot with your left hand (**note: if you're unsure about a limitation from a joint replacement or if your**

Toe-Stretching Devices

Your toes have been squished together for a long time, and even if you're consistent about stretching them a few times a day (or if you have a hip or knee replacement that prohibits you from the toe-stretching position), you can use a pair of toe-separating socks (like Foot Alignment Socks) or other toe separators (like Correct Toes, which you can even wear in your shoes if your shoes are sufficiently wide). Only use them for a few minutes at a time at first while your toes become accustomed to having some space between them. Eventually you may be able to wear them all day and night.

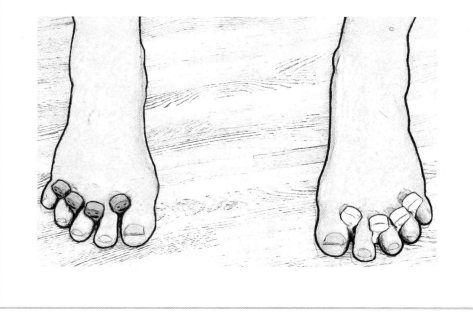

hips are too stiff to do this yet, see the options in the sidebar on page 37). Insert the fingers of your left hand between the toes of your right foot and hold for at least one minute. You're in control of this stretch: to increase it, push your fingers more deeply between the toes so that the webbing of your fingers and toes meet. To deepen even more, gently stretch your fingers apart, which will bring the toes with them. And of course, to

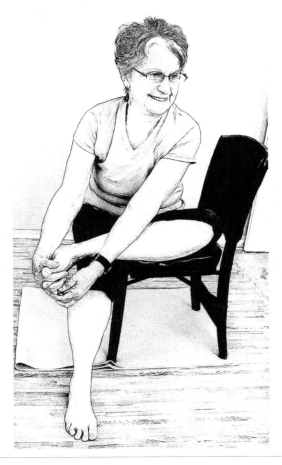

Tip from the Goldeners

Cold feet got you down? Warm up your toes with a toe massage. Sit on the floor or on a chair, in a position where you can reach all the toes on one foot, such as with one foot up on the opposite leg's thigh (mind any knee or hip replacements; for an exercise that will make this easier for you eventually, see page 132).

Grasp the big toe of the foot and pull it out, away from the pinkie. Using your hand, move the toe in large clockwise and counterclockwise motions. Continue these circular motions for up to thirty seconds on each toe, then repeat on the other foot. We've found that as the circulation is increased in our toes, they support us better while we exercise.

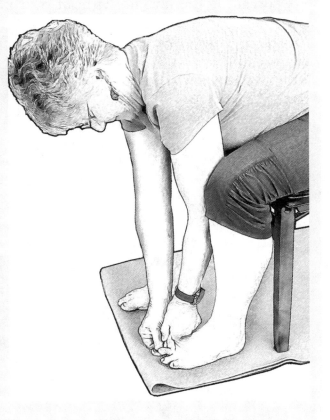

lessen it, do the reverse. Hold this for up to a minute or two, then switch to the other side, and repeat often throughout the day, preferably at least three times, until your toes stretch more easily.

Once you've stretched your toes with your hands, stand and try spreading them again without your hands, making sure your weight is shifted back over your heels (it's hard to spread them when your weight is bearing down on them). Try to make space between each toe, keeping all the toes flat on the ground. Are your toe-spreading muscles more responsive after a little bit of stretching?

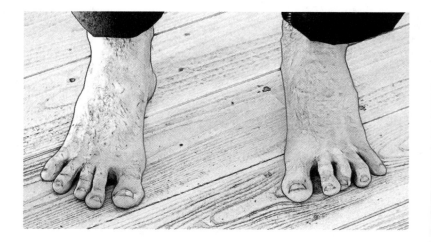

We lose the ability to spread our toes when we don't ever spread them. The good news is that the more you practice spreading and the more you work your toes apart with your hands, the better they'll be able to respond to the signals you're sending.

Repeat this exercise throughout the day, with or without shoes (and you'll know whether your shoes are too narrow if you can't do this exercise while wearing them).

Tip from the Goldeners

Choose a time of day or a location to do these toe exercises regularly. Remind yourself by posting a sticky note—"toe exercises!"—on your bathroom mirror, at the kitchen sink, or at your desk. Someplace that, when you see it, you'll be able to do the exercises right then.

TOE LIFTS

It's easier to lift all your toes at once than one at a time, but the ability to lift them separately means you're in better control of your feet. To test your ability to use your toe muscles individually, try lifting just your big toes while keeping the other eight toes on the ground.

Then, try lifting just the big toe on the left foot, and then the right.

Work to lift each big toe straight upward, rather than letting it veer sideways (toward the pinkie toe).

After you've mastered lifting your big toes, try lifting first them and then the second toe of each foot, making sure to keep the balls of your feet on the floor. Then lift the third, fourth, and fifth toes. Once all the toes are lifted, put them back down one by one. Then try this again, but one foot at a time.

If you're unable to lift your toes one toe at a time, don't worry! Keep working on toe spreading and lifting, and address your footwear choices. Eventually, your toes will start listening.

When you're finished with all this toe work, stretch them out with the Top of the Foot Stretch.

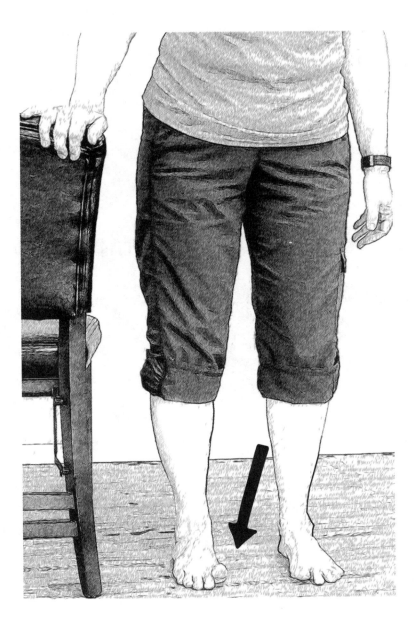

Barefoot-Friendly Floor Space

One of the reasons thick soles are recommended is because many of us have lost the ability to sense things with our feet, and may inadvertently step on something sharp enough to harm them. However, that puts us in a pickle—in order to redevelop our feet's sense, we need to go unshod and make them healthier, which then puts our feet at risk. The solution is to create a barefoot-friendly floor space.

- Vacuum an area you want to keep clear to make sure you don't step on any sharp debris (think pins, needles, etc.).

- For an extra layer of protection, roll out a thick towel or yoga mat over the area you've vacuumed.

- If your feet are very sensitive, double up on floor coverings—put a mat over a carpet, or layer a blanket or many towels for cushioning.

- Any time you're going to your barefoot space, do another visual check for any items you don't want to step on.

FOOTWEAR

My book *Simple Steps to Foot Pain Relief* is all about shoes, feet, and foot pain, because feet and what we put them in are complex. But here are some things, briefly, to consider about shoes.

As I mentioned earlier, shoes are a kind of cast on our feet. But there are some shoes that offer more movement to your feet and the rest of the body. If you've been casted in your shoes for a long time and want to switch to more body-friendly shoes, it's important to transition slowly for your foot health. Here are the elements you should look for in a shoe:

- **WIDE TOE BOX.** This is the part of the shoe that houses the front of your foot, and it's very narrow in most conventional footwear. (To see how narrow yours is compared to your foot, trace the outline of your shoe on a piece of paper, then place your bare foot in the same position and trace it. If the outline of your foot goes beyond the outline of your shoe, you're being squished every time you put those shoes on! And you should really be able to spread your toes wide in your shoes!) Choose shoes with room for you to spread your toes freely.

- **MINIMAL HEEL.** Any elevation at all in a shoe, whether it's a stiletto or a running shoe or a men's business shoe, changes the alignment of your body. You've just read why it's best to keep your weight back over the heels (and off the toes), but you can't shift your weight back when there's a heel constantly shifting it forward. It can take a year or even two to transition to less heel lift. Start with the exercises in the book and look for a slightly lower-heeled shoe, do the exercises more, and gradually increase the amount of time you spend in lower heels. Eventually you can transition to completely flat shoes and your muscles will be strong enough to support you.

- **FLEXIBLE SOLE.** The many bones, joints, and muscles in your feet need to move to stay healthy and strong, but most shoes are too stiff to allow your foot to change shape at all. Find a flexible shoe that allows for the most movement possible. Try twisting and bending the shoe to see how easily it moves. The more it does, the more your foot-parts will be able to move inside it.

- **FIXED UPPER.** Clogs, mules, and other slip-on shoes may seem like a safer option—no having to bend over or balance to tie them on—but in order to keep them on, you need to clench your toes. This can result in stiff and shortened muscles in the toes and ankles. Choose shoes that securely connect the upper portion of the shoe to the lower and that stay on your feet without you having to tense your body to keep them on.

- **NO TOE SPRING.** Toe spring is the upward curve of the toe portion of a shoe. Some shoes, particularly athletic shoes, have a great amount of toe spring, which can constantly force your toes upward. Find a shoe that lets your toes lie naturally.

Joyce Says

Since moving differently I've noticed the biggest change in my feet and knees.

After a lifetime of being squished, my feet are widening out and my toes are spreading. The top of my foot is flattening, and broadening, and bunions on both of my feet are gradually receding. My toes used to have humps at the joints like inchworms, but they're slowly straightening. I can lift and lower each of the toes of each foot individually.

My knees have lost the majority of the fluid retention initially caused by injuries twenty years ago, when I could hardly walk more than a block or two and some days not at all. In the past nine years I have restored enough mobility and strength in my feet, knees, and hips to sustain walks from one to three miles doing daily errands. I have the mobility to go freely and joyfully up and down the stairs to my apartment and to go hiking with friends in the hills and mountains and at the beach two or three times weekly. It is indeed a blessing to be alive, well, and walking at nearly eighty years young.

CHAPTER 2

BALANCE, STABILITY, AND GETTING OVER THE FEAR OF FALLING

Falls don't "just happen," and people don't fall because they get older.

—NIH Senior Health website

I can't remember first learning to walk with balance—I was only a year old—but I can tell you that my life changed dramatically after I mastered that skill. Balance is vital at any age, and although it seems like goldeners are special in that they really need to work on their balance, I can tell you from working with thousands of people that many, of all ages, aren't really walking in an efficient, balanced way. Age isn't solely respon-sible for a dramatic loss of balance—the problem is more a sedentary lifestyle where you haven't practiced balance in a long time. That all said, the consequences of falling are greater once you pass the bouncy-tissue age of two, and so it's no wonder many goldeners carry with them a fear of falling that permeates all of their movement decisions.

A few years ago I visited Taos Pueblo in New Mexico. On a tour I learned that the original buildings had no doors—and that tribal members of all ages (thought to be up to fifty or sixty) had to get into their home by climbing up a ladder to the roof and then down another ladder into the dwelling. While they didn't live as long as many of us do now, they maintained the ability to climb ladders with ease their entire lifespan. And that's when I started to merge my understanding of exercise science with my understanding of anthropology—getting up and down a ladder is made more challenging simply by the fact that we rarely use ladders and that the moves we do with confidence are simply the moves that we do multiple times a day. Thus, it's easy to see how one could mistake the wobbliness that comes from many decades of very little movement with the accumulation of the decades themselves.

Despite "age" seeming to be the obvious cause of so many falls, age itself isn't a maker of falls, according to the National Institutes of Health. The Centers for Disease Control and Prevention suggests that one first address the following movement-related risks:

- A sedentary lifestyle
- Lower-body weakness
- Foot problems
- Gait and balance difficulties

As my good friends and co-contributors to this book will tell you, their experience of muscular weakness was not a result of aging so much as a result of decreased movement over a number of years. We live in an age of technology. Technology that's been slowly increasing in scope and reducing our needs for movement. It's very likely that the instability you are feeling is not due to your age, but to how long you *haven't* been challenging your balance.

ENTER FEAR OF FALLING

Another risk factor for falling is the *fear* of falling. Meaning that simply being afraid of a fall (or its imagined aftermath) is enough to change the way we move.

If you've experienced a fall, it's natural to be wary of another.

 Joyce Says

I was sixty-eight when I realized I no longer felt safe on a ladder picking oranges from our orange tree. I didn't believe it at first, but on repeated attempts, I could not change the feeling of unsteadiness and fear when I attempted to mount the ladder beyond the first or second rung. The loss of my sense of balance was unmistakable. I felt a heavy resignation and thought to myself, "Oh, this is what it's like to age."

> **People who hadn't fallen, but reported a fear of falling, were more likely to fall in the future.**

Still, studies done over a two-year period found that while a feeling of unsteadiness coupled with previous falls was a large contributor to fear, 18 percent of the "fearful" group had a large fear of falling without having fallen before (Lach 2005).

Researchers, trying to determine whether a fall creates fear or fear creates a fall, discovered that people who hadn't fallen, but reported a fear of falling, were more likely to fall in the future—despite the fact that they had decreased their activity level to reduce the opportunity for a fall (Friedman et al. 2002).

This is a sample of a wide body of work demonstrating that fear in itself is a risk factor for falling. The next question is, of course, why? Or perhaps more pertinently, how?

There is a generalization we can make about goldeners' gait—that it becomes a slow, careful shuffle, easily recognized. What may come as a surprise is that research shows this way of walking—short stride lengths, shuffling feet, and low speed—is for the most part without a mechanical cause; it involves self-induced adjustments (Herman et al. 2005). In fact, gait disorders of this kind—in healthy seniors with no disease, previous falls, or weaker muscles than their counterparts—were largely a response to fear alone.

Of course, it's perfectly natural to change how you walk in response to a fear of falling. When I moved from sunny California to my first icy Washington winter, I adopted a very similar way of moving to the one described above. I walked more slowly. I turned my feet out, bent my knees a bit to lower my center of gravity, and I started shuffling. When I recently paid attention to how I walked in a situation where I felt vulnerable to a fall, I noticed it wasn't only my lower half adjusting. My neck and shoulders stiffened. My hands stiffened too, and so did my face. Anyone who's walked over a slippery surface or spent any time on the ice or snow has likely altered their movement patterns to prevent a fall; these changes are a natural

It's Not the Fall, It's the Faller

A fall is not an issue in and of itself. Humans fall all the time without equal penalty. The impact of a fall has more to do with the state of the body doing the falling—the interface between a body and a particular surface. Robust tissues—supple muscles and ligaments, strong bones, and the ability to quickly adjust your shape—hold the potential to reduce the impact of a fall.

For this reason I suggest improving not only your balance and stability, but also your joint mobility, muscle mass, and bone density. This seems like it will take a lot of different exercises, but here's the good news: The exercise program in this book addresses *all of these at once*. I don't only want you to learn to balance on one leg; I want you to do it in a way that uses the muscles in the hip, which will then pull on bones of your hip, signaling "grow stronger." If it seems like I'm getting a little nitpicky in my form requirements for each exercise, it is only because this form targets multiple issues at once, so that many issues can be improved from the same set of exercises.

response to fear. But I want you to consider this for a moment: We've essentially mislabeled "scared gait" as "senior gait."

The way we walk has a profound impact on the muscles used while walking and vice versa. When you shuffle, you're not moving your ankles much, and so the muscles that facilitate ankle movement adapt by stiffening. Now your ankles can't move when you need them to. When you bend your knees slightly all the time to keep your body mass low, you work the muscles down the front of the leg a lot, but you also reduce the work of the hips, giving you tight thigh muscles, but weak and stiff hips and, quite possibly, lower bone mass in the hips as well.

Adjusting the way you walk to reduce your fall risk in times of actual increased risk can serve you well. But "walking afraid" with every step doesn't, in the end, protect you from falls. It weakens your body in ways that actually make you *more* susceptible to falls in the long run.

The key to reducing your risk of falling is to strengthen your body in a way that gives you a confident gait, which in turn strengthens your body even more, and so on.

Practicing a Fall

The greatest fear of all may be fear of the unknown, and since after childhood we fall so infrequently, falling is a big unknown for us. Because we're afraid and have so little experience with falling, we tend to tense up rather than relaxing when we *do* fall, which changes the forces created by a fall.

A goldener named Elliott Royce set out to change that. At the age of ninety-five, he was falling five times a day—on purpose. Just as professional athletes practice drills over and over until their movements are almost reflexive, Royce intentionally fell onto an air mattress repeatedly to train his body to fall in a way that would reduce the impact of the fall on his body. From a *StarTribune* article about his method:

> "The secret to falling safely is three words: bend, twist, roll," he said.
>
> As you start to fall, bend your knees in the direction you are falling and twist at the waist, turning your shoulders away from the fall. That will change the point of impact. Instead of one spot on your hip taking the entire brunt of the fall, the force will be spread out along the length of your leg, thigh and pelvis. When you hit the ground, roll to further dissipate the force of the impact." (Strickler 2015)

Royce's approach to aligning his fall, which he taught to other goldeners, makes sense. When he had real falls—and he did—his body automatically responded in a protective way. Being leery of a fall is different from being afraid of one. Put your fear to rest by building a more robust structure and approach a physical therapist or movement teacher to help you institute your own "safe falling" practice.

YOU ARE HOW YOU WALK

More stable walking begins with your feet, which we began working on in chapter 1. After you've warmed up the toes and bones within the feet, it's time to address the ankles.

Stable walking requires a lot of ankle mobility. The stiffer your ankles, the more you have to either shuffle or lift your entire foot away from the ground at the hip—both of which leave you more vulnerable to falls. Walking heel-toe allows you to transfer your weight from foot to foot in a more controlled manner, and it keeps your calf muscles supple and strong.

FEET FORWARD

In order to fully use your ankles while walking, your feet need to point forward, more like tires on a car, and less out to the sides like a duck. Align the outside edge of each foot with a straight edge, like a book or the seam of a carpet. When you straighten your feet, you'll likely feel your knees and hips turn as well (see pages 76–78 for an additional step if you're feeling knock-kneed). You'll be using this forward foot position for most exercises in this book and can start working it into your walk. **DON'T force your feet forward while walking,** but instead pay attention to just how far your feet turn out and shoot for slightly less when you walk (an adjustment that's shown to decrease the angles of the knee associated with knee osteoarthritis) (Shull et al. 2013).

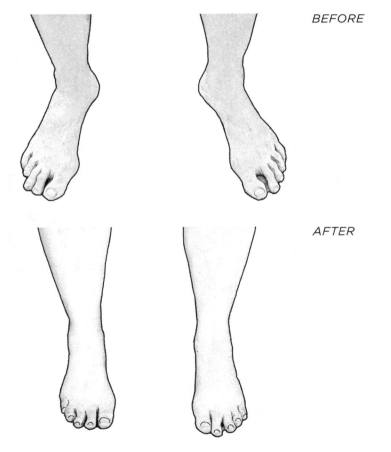

BEFORE

AFTER

CALF STRETCHES

The calf muscles are what often limit full motion of your ankle. These exercises are an excellent way to address tight calves!

CALF STRETCH #1

The first Calf Stretch targets the calf muscle that runs behind the knees, which is why you need to keep the knee straight on the stretching leg. To bend it is to diminish the stretch.

With a wall or chair close by for balance assistance, place a thick folded and rolled towel (or a rolled yoga mat) on the floor in front of you. Step onto the towel with a bare or socked foot, placing the ball of the foot on the top of the towel and keeping your heel on the floor.

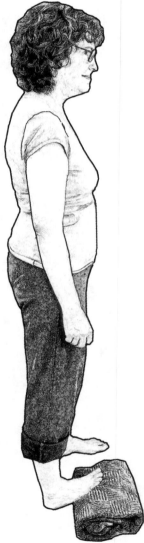

Adjust the foot so that it points straight forward, and slowly straighten your stretching leg.

Keeping your body upright (try not to lean forward with your torso), step forward with the opposite foot.

The tighter your lower leg, the harder it will be to step in front of your stretching leg. It's common to keep the non-stretching leg behind the towel at first. If you're leaning forward, finding you need to bend your knees, or losing your balance, shorten your stepping distance.

If you want to make the move more advanced, use a half foam roller instead of a rolled towel.

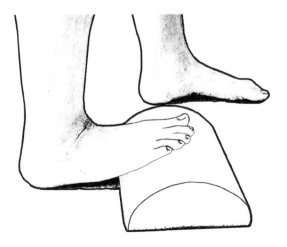

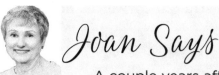

Joan Says

A couple years after starting to do the Calf Stretch at least twice a day, morning and night, I noticed an interesting change in my hiking. Previously when I hiked uphill, I usually landed on the ball of my front foot because I couldn't put my heel down. After lots of Calf Stretch practice, the range of motion in my ankles increased until I could land on my heels as I stepped uphill. This changed the muscles I was using to go uphill from my quads (on the fronts of my thighs) to those on my backside (hamstrings and butt). Katy had said using the hamstrings and glutes while walking (she calls it a "posterior push-off") could help build a butt or retrieve one that was disappearing. And she was right! That is exactly what has happened to me. My co-authors and others who have known me for a while have commented over these past several years about the noticeable development of my gluteal muscles. In addition to moving with better strength and stability, I'm appreciating how I firmly fill out the back pockets of my pants.

CALF STRETCH #2

This second Calf Stretch targets the deeper muscle in the calf group—the soleus—that affects the mobility between the foot and the shin. You get to bend your knee for this one!

Beginning in the position of Calf Stretch #1, bend the knee of the foot on the rolled towel, pushing it slightly forward as you press that same heel toward the ground.

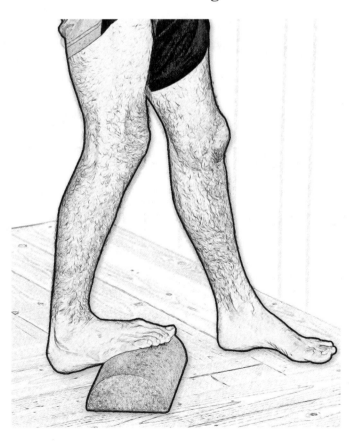

Both calf exercises are designed to improve the ease of ankle movement when walking on flat ground *and* uphill.

Moving well requires the ability to walk comfortably, which requires balance, which depends heavily on the strength of a particular group of muscles: those of the lateral hip—which brings us to our next chapter.

 Lora Says

I've been in love with my half foam roller from the start. I had immediate success with the disappearance of restless leg syndrome, and as the half foam roller was my only new exercise prop at the time, I credited the dome with that miracle. After that first movement session I began a now seven-year habit of keeping a half foam roller in my kitchen. I have four-course mornings of breakfast, mind-strengthening games, keeping up with current events, and doing the Calf Stretch—it all keeps me feeling well nourished!

Joyce Says
Within a few years of starting to work with Katy, I once again was able to climb ladders and step ladders without fear. It was a marvelous feeling of personal power that I am grateful for. In the past few years, I have realized that once again I can climb stairs, go down stairs, climb mountains, go down mountains, skip, hop, jump, and leap for fun and also when I need to. I can squat, sit on the floor with comfort, sleep on the floor with comfort, kneel, hang from trees, swing on bars. These are all movements I took for granted as a child and up until somewhere in midlife, when these were no longer a part of my movement patterns.

CHAPTER 3
SUPER-STRONG HIPS AND SINGLE-LEGGED BALANCE

Super-strong hips, much like this book, start with the feet. Not only the mobility of the feet, but also how you stack your body over them. You've already learned how to back your hips up and keep your weight off the front of your feet. The reason the front of your feet push so hard into the ground when your hips jut forward is they're trying to keep you from falling forward. Standing with your hips out in front of you is sort of like falling while you're standing! Thus, backing up your hips (see page 28 for a reminder) is not only for your feet or even for your hips—it is also a fast way to reduce any tendency to fall. Easy, right?

Strong hips and stability go hand in hand. One simple thing you can do to start improving your balance and to give your lateral hip muscles more of a chance to strengthen is to make small adjustments to how you stand in everyday life. As you actively call on new positioning, the muscles from the top of your head to the bottom of your feet start to support you in a subtle yet constant way. Over time, new postures can bring about new muscle mass specific to your new stance, eventually allowing you to relax and be more supported. Below are some stance guidelines for you to work toward. **Note**: All of the exercises and stances in this chapter are to be done in bare or socked feet, or completely flat shoes—wearing a heel of any height can make many of these movements impossible.

FEET PELVIS-WIDTH APART

The width of your stance and gait pattern matters. Walking with your feet too close together or too wide apart can affect your stability and which muscles you use when you walk. There are times when you have to go wide or narrow due to the terrain over which you're walking, but when you're standing

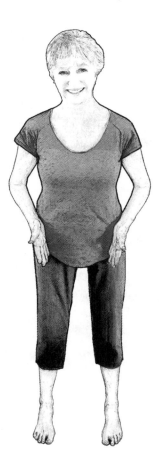

around, stand with your feet pelvis-width apart, weight centered between the two. This alignment not only gives you a solid base, but will also help you recruit the muscles of the hips once you start walking.

LEGS VERTICAL

The activation of your lateral hip muscles (see page 83 for a picture) depends on the geometry of your lower body. A tendency to slightly bend the knees can disable these muscles, and so to better turn on the lateral hip muscles, this tendency needs addressing first.

After you've shifted your weight back, straighten your knees (or, if you tend to hyperextend your knees, bend them a tad) until they fall directly between your hips and ankle joints in a vertical line. A mirror and a plumb line will help you find this position, as will the next alignment tip.

BEFORE   *AFTER*

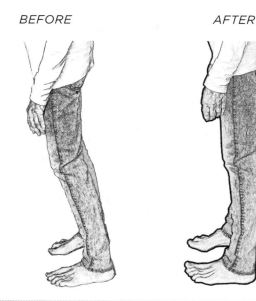

RELAXED KNEECAPS

If you've been thrusting your hips forward and slightly bending your knees for decades, your quadriceps—the muscles on the front of your thighs that attach to your kneecaps—have been doing the bulk of the work to keep you from tumbling forward. It's good that you haven't been tumbling forward, but all that tension pulls the bone of the kneecap (also known as the patella) deep into the knee joint, where it can slowly rub against the tissues below.

Relaxing your quads lowers and decreases the interaction between the patella and your knee joint, and it also allows other muscles on the sides and backs of your thigh to participate better. Eventually you'll be able to relax the kneecaps while standing, but first, try it seated.

Sit at the front of a chair with your legs straight ahead of you and heels resting on the floor. Your kneecaps can't relax if your knees are bent, so first things first, allow the legs to straighten all the way. If you've been bracing sore or stiff knees, this can

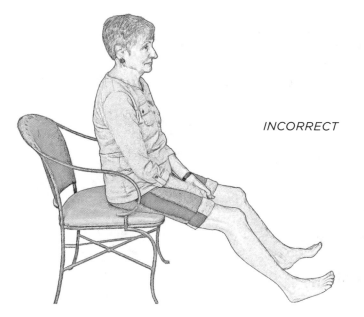

INCORRECT

take a bit of time. If you're using a mirror, sit so you can see your legs from the side, where a slightly bent knee is more visible. Once your legs are straight, relax your quad muscles. This will result in a visible lowering of your kneecaps toward your ankles.

Once you can relax your kneecaps sitting, try it more upright. Using a wall to support your hips (see image page 74), place your feet about twelve to eighteen inches out from the wall, and straighten your legs. Try lifting and lowering the kneecaps in that position.

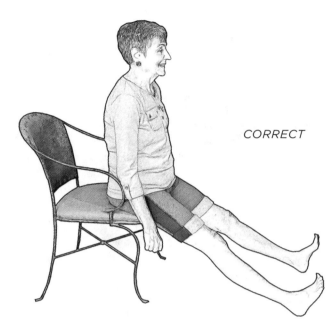

CORRECT

Now try it standing fully upright. (See image page 75.) This is the most challenging because you might be so used to holding your weight with slightly bent knees that once the chair and wall are gone, you go back to your old habit. To set yourself up, stand in front of a mirror with your weight shifted back over your heels, and straighten your legs. Can you release your knee-caps now?

If not, go back to where you last could and keep working on it! The skill will come eventually, especially if you're regularly practicing your stance alignment and choosing to wear shoes that allow you to keep your weight shifted back.

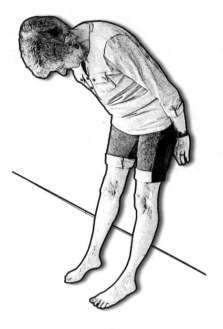

If you've had gripping tension in your quadriceps for decades and decades, you may have to remind your kneecaps to lower hundreds of times a day as you go about your daily life. This is fine! Every time you think about it, you're bringing awareness to a subconscious habit, and every time you adjust you're moving your knees differently than before.

Tip from the Goldeners

To release your kneecaps, start by contracting them, then think *release*. If there is no movement, gently brush your fingers over your kneecaps to bring sensory awareness to the muscles. Kneecap release can be difficult as most of us chronically contract our quadriceps, locking the kneecaps. The motor skill to release this hold may be asleep.

QUADS TENSE, KNEECAPS PULLED UP   QUADS RELAXED, KNEECAPS DOWN

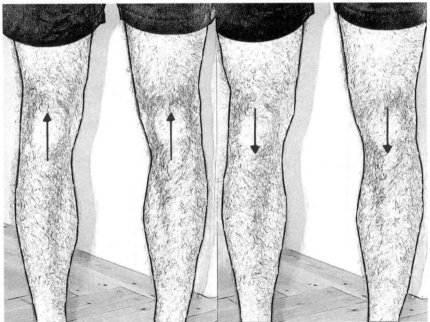

NEUTRAL KNEE-PITS

Stand with your legs bare and your back to a mirror. Turn your head or bend forward to look at the back of your knees; you'll see two dents on each leg that mark the tendons of your hamstring muscles—I call these your "knee-pits." Ideally, all

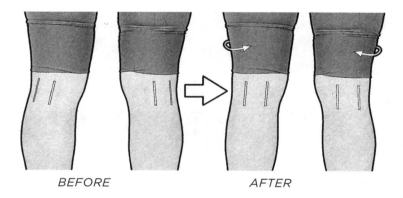

BEFORE　　　　　*AFTER*

four dents should align directly behind you, as your feet point straight ahead. This means that your ankles and knees can both hinge in the plane you are walking along, which is typically straight ahead.

In most cases, because of how we've moved or not moved our bodies, these lines no longer line up. To start working on getting your knee and ankle joints to line up, rotate your thighs

Knee-friendly External Rotation

Because our feet are stiff, when you first start rotating your thighs it will be almost impossible to keep the soles of your feet on the ground. **Do not force your feet to stay down when externally rotating your thighs—this can strain your knees.** Let the inner edges of your feet lift so you roll up on the outside of your feet as you turn your thighs. Your feet will need to do this less over time if you're regularly practicing your foot-mobilizing exercises!

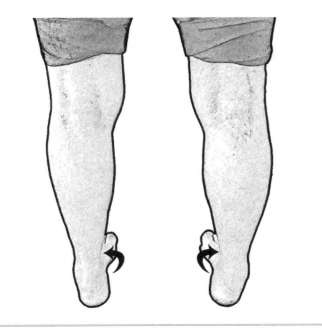

to bring all four lines to a neutral position (typically this means you'll rotate the fronts of your thighs away from each other, allowing the instep of your feet to lift; if you try to keep your feet flat, you can strain your knees—see sidebar above).

It's unlikely that your right and left leg will be rotating the same amount. The turnout of our feet is rarely symmetrical, which means the correction won't be either (i.e., you might have to turn your left thigh more or less than the right to line up all knee-pit lines).

OBSERVE YOUR BALANCE

When we don't move very often, our body loses the ability to make rapid adjustments to our rapidly changing position. And so, when we stand up after long bouts of sitting, our bodies are out of practice as to what to do.

We all feel a little wobbly on one leg, but sometimes we even feel wobbly on two legs. This is why I like to start working on balance with both feet firmly on the ground.

Line up your stance (straight feet, straight legs, hips over heels, etc.). **Lightly touching a wall or chair**, close your eyes and observe how you feel. Do you feel like your body is swaying to and fro while you're standing on two feet?

Joan Says

In my first session with Katy, she showed me how to improve my stance: feet pointing forward, hip-width apart, and weight back in my heels. I felt pigeon-toed and unbalanced, and thought I looked like a cowboy with such a wide stance. She showed me how my rib thrust was compressing my low back (which always used to hurt) and explained how my habits of tucking my pelvis and sucking in my abdomen were contributing to my weak abs, constipation, and pelvic prolapse. In that session, I discovered that I was a rib-thruster, butt-tucker, and ab-sucker. And so, my journey began.

A year before, in 2008, I had been scheduled for pelvic reconstructive surgery to "correct" the prolapse. To date, surgery has been unnecessary and my pelvic floor muscles are improving. I hike for miles in barefoot shoes. And my chronic, lifetime constipation was permanently resolved in 2012, as a direct result of this work. It all started with the stance for me!

Step one in restoring your balance is to spend five to six minutes a day practicing "stilling" yourself. Repeat this exercise, but instead of observing your wobbliness, try to steady yourself without tensing. Think "relaxed stability," not "stiff statue."

Once you're more balanced on two legs, you can move to one.

First, observe. **Holding lightly on to a wall or chair,** try standing on one leg. Either leg is fine. See what it takes for you to keep your balance. Are your toes gripping? Is your leg tensed? Knee bent? Are you hanging on to the wall or a chair? Are you wobbling? Is your pelvis drifting out in front of you? How long were you able to stay stable on one foot?

After you've observed, next on the list is practice. Can you relax your toes? Back your hips over your heels? Straighten your knees without locking them (i.e., pulling up your kneecaps)? Can you drop your shoulders? Breathe in a relaxed way? As you remove unnecessary reactions—body geometries and muscle tensions that aren't required to keep you on a single leg—you'll be more practiced in recruiting the necessary parts that allow you to move in a fluid balance. Again, on one leg (and really whenever you're moving) you want relaxed stability and not stiff statue.

Standing on one leg can feel like a circus trick, but here's the thing: Walking is essentially a bout of single-leg balance

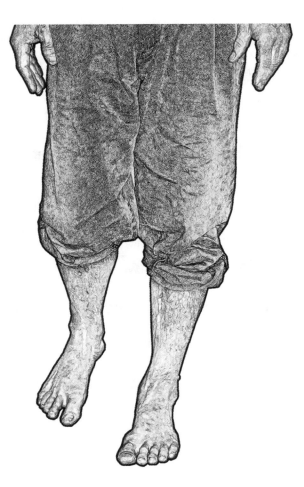

followed by another and another, and so on. When you're on a

single leg, the bone and lateral hip muscles of this one leg must

be strong enough to carry the weight of the entire body. When

your hip muscles aren't strong enough, you're forced to compen-

sate by shortening your stride (to decrease the amount of time your one hip is carrying the body) or walking with a shuffle (where you never actually stand on a single leg).

If you're using strong hip muscles to lift your left leg, the muscles down the outside of your right hip pull the right side of the pelvis slightly downward, which slightly lifts the left side. This lift gives the left leg room to swing through, clearing the ground easily. When the hip muscles work in this way, not only is motion controlled throughout the gait cycle—i.e., the walker has more balance—but also the hip bones are better challenged, keeping them stronger and less susceptible to a fracture in the event of a fall. It's a cycle: the stronger your walking muscles, the more stable your walk, which in turn continues to strengthen your body.

Ideally, your lateral hip muscles should have the strength and endurance to elevate and maintain the position of the floating leg. Unfortunately, many people (of all ages) are lacking strong enough hip musculature, and their gait is suffering. What should be walking is just a series of quick, consecutive falls.

The Lateral Hip Muscles

Put your right hand on your hip and slide it down to the top of your leg. You've just passed over your lateral hip muscles (used in the Pelvic List, page 85). These muscles are the tensor fasciae latae, gluteus medius, and gluteus minimus.

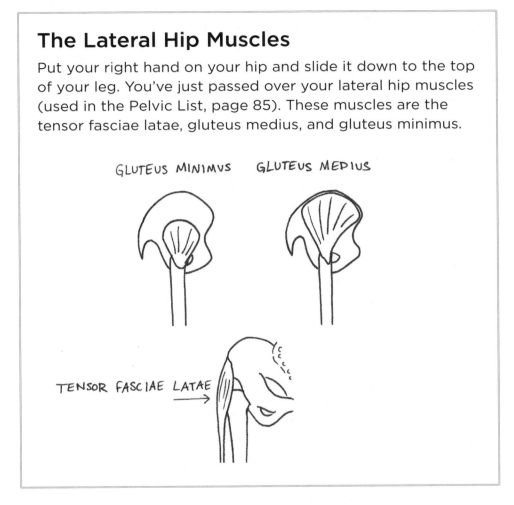

GLUTEUS MINIMUS   GLUTEUS MEDIUS

TENSOR FASCIAE LATAE →

There are a lot of people who can ride a bicycle without it falling over, but very few can sit on an unmoving bike (with their feet off the ground) without it falling. Why? Continuous forward movement masks balance deficiencies. And just as the cyclist makes super-fast corrections to a thousand invisible almost-falls, "walking" with a body weakened by modern living is actually just one controlled fall after another.

 Joyce Says

I didn't believe Katy when she first said I was falling and not walking. I could walk at a good clip! I was an avid hiker and backpacker for most of my life. Maybe other folks were falling, but not me.

It took many months for me to check out my walk, looking for signs of "falling." As I became attuned to the way I walked, sure enough, I was falling forward, landing with a thud with each foot's "fall" on the ground. Once I got it, I began the journey of awareness, correction, exercises, and practice. I needed all of these to finally be able to support my weight on one leg. I am a better walker now, though I still have a way to go. My ultimate goal is to be able to walk with such good balance that I can put my foot down silently exactly where I want it to go.

THE PELVIC LIST

The Pelvic List is an exercise that is designed specifically to target the muscles you need to be able to stand strongly on a single leg.

Holding lightly on to a wall or chair, stand with both your feet forward, ankles positioned at pelvic width. Shift your weight back over your heels and find your vertical leg. Place your right hand on your right hip and, using the muscles on the outside of the right hip, bring the right side of your pelvis down toward the floor. This downward action will result in your left foot lifting away from the ground. Check to make sure you're not bending either knee. (Note that if your left foot doesn't clear the ground, that's okay; keep practicing engaging these muscles until it does).

Observe. Is your standing ankle wobbling or your floating foot touching down periodically? Is your pelvis drifting forward, or are your knees bending? Can you let go, or do you need to hold on to something in order to stay balanced? These would all be signs that your lateral hip muscles are not fully engaging when you're walking—meaning, your walk is more falling than it needs to be. This is good news, though. It means that as your hips strengthen, your need for the compensations will lessen.

After the Calf Stretch, the Pelvic List is my favorite corrective for the improvement it offers. It's also a corrective that can fit easily into your daily movement. At first you'll be doing it as an exercise, but soon you can do it with each step—every step you take is an opportunity to put more hip into it. When you're

Shelah Says

My favorite corrective exercise is the Pelvic List. For a number of years I have traveled several times a year to foreign countries on craft or fiber-related trips. Before changing how I moved, I would fall at least once on each trip, usually on the street or steps. After some time doing classes with Katy, I stopped falling. Now, I generally feel quite confident on uneven surfaces: narrow bridges (if they aren't too high), cobblestone streets, etc. My balance has improved dramatically. And the Pelvic List is portable too; no equipment required. I take it with me every time I travel!

practicing the Pelvic List as an exercise, watch for cheats: You can achieve the look of this exercise by *lifting* the pelvis using the lower back of the floating side (as opposed to *pulling down* with the hip of the standing leg). To remedy, touch the lateral hip of your standing leg to remind yourself, "this is the working part."

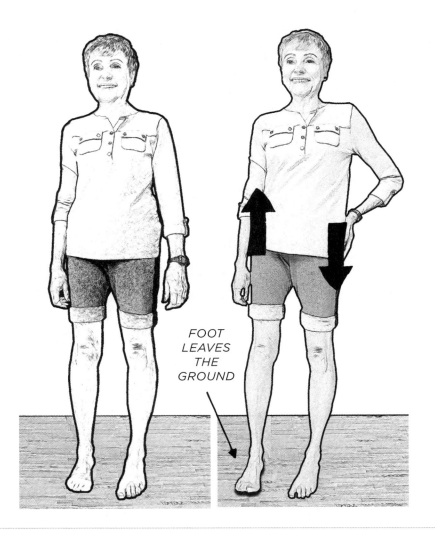

FOOT LEAVES THE GROUND

CHAPTER 4
WALKING

The more you move, the more you strengthen your body, thus the more you feel comfortable with your body, which in turn helps you move more, which makes you even more body-confident...you see how this works?

Walking, as mundane as it may seem, is the backbone of most functional tasks. It's also a great way to interact with others and the natural world around you, and it's free! Learning to move more involves learning to walk more. The postural adjustments and corrective exercises in this book, even the ones for the head and shoulders (coming up), are to help you strengthen often-neglected areas of the body so that you become more competent and confident as you walk.

KEEPING FORM

You've already learned ways to adjust your form while standing and exercising, many of which can be integrated into your walk for better balance and stability. Add the following as you feel comfortable. You'll likely find focusing on one at a time easiest, but as your body strengthens, many of these will begin to occur naturally.

- **FEET FORWARD.** If you have a lot of turnout, turn your feet in a small amount at first; see page 58–59 for details.

- **WEIGHT BACK ON YOUR HEELS.** Make sure your hips don't enter the room before you do! See page 28 for details.

- **CENTER YOUR PELVIS.** There are bony protrusions of your pelvis (side view labeled page 91) that are easy to use to figure out how you're positioned. After adjusting your feet and legs as noted above, move the pelvis until the ASIS (anterior superior iliac spines—those pointy parts on the front of your pelvis) and pubic symphysis line up on a vertical plane together. For many,

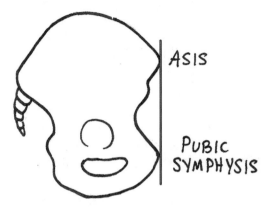

this will mean *untucking* your pelvis to tip the front of the pelvis forward. If you have been tucking for some time, it's normal to feel like your bum is sticking out at first, but that's fine! Just as backing your hips up loads your hip bones and muscles more, keeping your pelvis neutral when standing, walking, and carrying helps your hips, spine, core, and pelvic floor respond to your weight most effectively.

- **CENTER YOUR RIBCAGE.** To keep your ribcage centered, line your bottom front ribs up on the same plane as the ASIS and pubic symphysis. Your core muscles run between your pelvis and ribcage. When your skeleton is stacked while standing and carrying, your trunk muscles can respond to your weight (and the weight of what you're carrying) most effectively. Allowing your ribcage to center will reveal the true curvature in your upper back. If you find yourself staring straight at the ground, see the next step!

• **HEAD RAMPED.** Without lifting it, slide your chin back until your ears align over your shoulders, keeping the back of your neck long (you'll know you're in position when you have at least two extra chins). This mobilizes your upper spine and will start decreasing some of that curvature you revealed when you centered your ribcage.

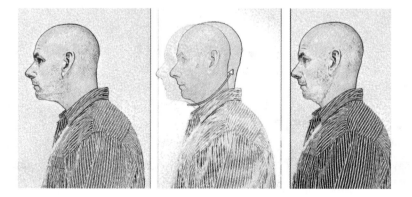

DYNAMIC AGING

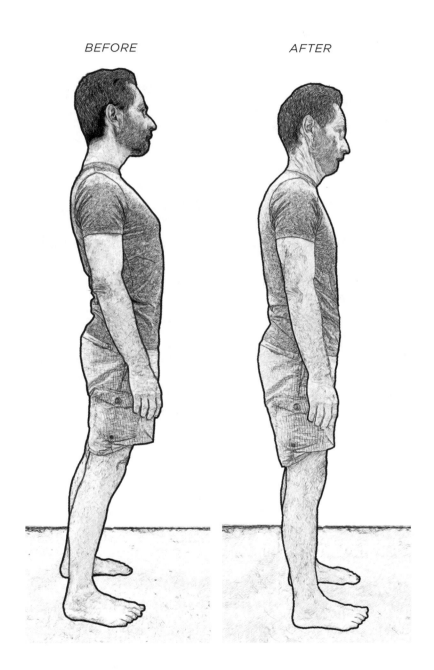

BEFORE

AFTER

Once you find yourself walking with more ease, you can increase the challenge of your walk in the following ways:

INCREASE YOUR MILEAGE

Try adding a small amount of distance to your walk every day. If you can walk half a mile right now, extend your walk by five or ten minutes. Gradually build up your mileage, increasing it incrementally. Some people like to use a pedometer to track their progress; others prefer to watch the clock, or just pay attention to the distance they've covered. Soon you'll be able to feel when you've passed your "normal" distance and you're pushing yourself just a little to walk farther.

INCREASE THE FREQUENCY OF YOUR WALK

Bear in mind that you don't have to do all your walking at once. In fact, walking in chunks is beneficial in that it gets you up and out multiple times throughout the day—something that's been shown to change the state of your arteries. For example, taking three one-mile walks in a day can be more beneficial to your health than taking one three-mile walk, especially if you spend most of the rest of the day sitting. That all said, walking for a continuous hour keeps up your ability to do so. So in the interest of moving more, keep that hour walk and add a few ten-to-fifteen-minute walks here and there!

STIMULATE YOUR BRAIN BY CHANGING YOUR ROUTE

An easy way to keep your brain active is to surprise it. This can be as simple as walking a different route from usual, so your mind has to sit up and take notice. Even reversing your usual route will perk up your awareness—and your body will have to move a little differently and as a result, strengthen a little differently.

ADD HILLS

Hills use your muscles and joints in different ways from walking over flat ground, so to never walk up and down hills, even small slopes, is to lose the strength and stamina to be able to do so. Seek out a few hills close to you—even a gently slop-

ing driveway in your neighborhood or a hill in a local park—

and walk up and down them a few times a week.

ADD "VITAMIN COMMUNITY"

One aspect of our physical health often overlooked is our

need for others (more on that on pages 177–179). In fact, one

of the reasons we want to move with greater ease in the first

place is that it allows us to go out into the world and be with

the people we love. Instead of doing your physical training in

isolation and then taking your "others time" in stillness, blend

---

Stairs Are Not Hills

Stairs can take you up and down, but the way you use your body on stairs is different from how you use your body on hills. The flatness and fixed height and length of each step forces your body to move in a particular way—often a way that can be hard on your knees. One way to take stairs with greater ease is to mind your form as you take them (see form tips on pages 127–131). Another is to condition your-self to hills—the more you do, the easier you'll be able to take the stairs!

---

the two and double the nutrition of your life! Get a walking buddy or start a walking group. It's much easier to increase your mileage, and more fun to change your route and add hills, if you're doing more than physical training. Chatting, laughing, and listening are hugely beneficial when it comes to connecting with others. A bonus: Having a scheduled walk with a friend or group adds accountability to your walking routine, which means you're likely to move more!

ADD "VITAMIN NATURE"

For a while now, research has shown that natural environments come with many healing benefits, but recent studies indicate that both green spaces and blue spaces (places with still or running water) are especially beneficial to goldeners (Finlay et al. 2015). Many use trips to nature to "escape it all" but goldeners in particular, it turns out, benefit from connecting back to it:

"We zoomed in to everyday life for seniors between the ages of 65 and 86. We discovered how a relatively mundane experience, such as hearing the sound of water or a bee buzzing among flowers, can have a tremendous impact on overall health," says Jessica Finlay, a former research assistant on [a study examining the effect of nature on the quality of life of goldeners]…and lead author of the paper. Finlay is now a doctoral candidate in geography and gerontology at the University of Minnesota, where she continues to investigate influences of the built environment [human-made structures and environments] on health and well-being in later life. "Accessibility to everyday green and blue spaces encourages seniors to simply get out the door. This in turn motivates them to be active physically, spiritually and socially, which can offset chronic illness, disability and isolation." (University of Minnesota 2015)

Search out a local park or pond you can walk to or around. Or, blend vitamin Nature with vitamin Community by joining your local Audubon Society chapter or other naturalist society that leads guided bird or plant identification walks. Or, simply meet your friends in the woods for some "forest bathing"—a term that refers to the researched health benefits that come from simply being around trees! (Park et al. 2009)

ADD "VITAMIN TEXTURE"

If you're concerned with the rambling (read: uneven) terrain found in natural spaces, train for them by adding vitamin Texture to your walk. After practicing your foot exercises and pillow train walking (see page 102 for the Pillow Train), start taking the grassy area beside the sidewalk for some gently varied movement in your feet and ankles. One exercise I've used for some time now is to put one foot up on a curb and one on the road and mindfully walk ten to twenty paces with my feet (and thus knees and hips) strengthening to this uneven form. The practice of walking on uneven and textured ground is what helps you be able to walk on uneven and textured ground!

WALK WITH PURPOSE

The very best way to make sure you walk every day is to make your walks useful. Begin to choose walking over other forms of transportation for your errands and appointments, and you'll find your mileage increasing naturally. If an errand is too far to walk, try parking farther away, or getting off the bus a few stops earlier, so you can incorporate walking for even longer-distance destinations.

OBSTACLES, OF COURSE

On one hand, obstacles increase your risk of falling. This is why so many approaches to "healthy aging" involve eliminating items from your home, like rugs that bunch and have high edges, and electrical cords. On the other hand, if you remove *all* the obstacles from your path, you also remove all the adaptations to them—the strength and speed necessary to respond accordingly. The ounce of prevention that is keeping a completely clear environment all the time might actually cause a fall later on, and

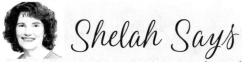

Shelah Says

My car was stolen about five years ago. After a few months I decided not to replace it. I still have a license and can drive if needed. But I found I could get around quite well without a car and an occasional taxi or Uber ride is less money and trouble than maintaining a car.

I live in the midtown area of Ventura. The transportation center, three grocery stores, and the shopping center are all less than a mile away. I got a wheeled shopping cart for carrying heavy items.

I also have many very kind friends and relatives and because I live in a central area, if need be I can almost always catch a ride to somewhere near my home.

And best of all, there is a bus stop two blocks from my house and because I am over seventy-five, I ride for free! The keys I have found are flexibility, planning ahead, and being grateful.

I know this works for me because I am able to walk comfortably several miles. Rather than being able to drive, being able to walk is my key to independence!

"safe movement" becomes limited to the confines of your home, which can encroach on your ability to get out and enjoy the rest of the world.

The solution to this dilemma is controlled obstacle training. I don't suggest you litter your home with objects that increase your risk of falling, but I *do* suggest you add obstacle training to your exercise routine. Here are a few easy and safe obstacles to begin with:

- **A TAPE "BALANCE BEAM."** Tape a line down the center of the floor for you to walk across as preliminary balance practice.

- **A "PILLOW TRAIN."** On a cleared surface, make a line of low, wide, soft objects, such as pillows, cushions, and folded towels and blankets, then practice walking across them in bare feet.

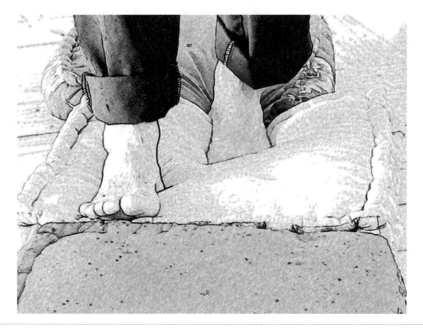

- **TALL OBSTACLES.** Once you've mastered the pillow train, add in some taller objects to step over. Begin with a small stack of books, then add taller objects as your agility increases.

- **SMALL OBSTACLES.** Place rounded, smooth rocks onto your pillow train and practice slowly walking on them. Placing them on the soft surfaces will lessen their impact at first. Eventually, try stepping on them on a yoga mat, carpet, and even hardwood floor. Transition slowly!

TAKE OFF YOUR SHOES

The shoes you wear affect how your muscles engage and how much they have to work. You can try each of the indoor exercises with your shoes off to increase the work your body has to do to balance you. Twenty-five percent of the muscles in your body reside from the ankle down. You can invite these neglected muscles to the balance party by removing over-stabilizing footwear and waking up your feet. To walk barefoot, make sure to clear the area of any sharp or potentially hazardous items, especially if you are experiencing any neuropathy in your feet. (For more foot-specific information and exercises, see chapter 1.)

KEEP IT LOOSE

Try to identify any muscles that are "helping" when they shouldn't be. Slight knee bending, toe gripping, and tensing the neck and shoulders are common reflexes when we feel unstable, but chronic practice of these motions eventually interferes with a healthy gait.

Consider this: The muscle patterns you develop to cope with a balance exercise reappear when you actually need to balance. If your toes grip when you're standing on one foot, for example, there is a good chance they grip during the balance phase of your gait cycle as well. This toe-gripping reduces the foot's ability to deal with new information, which leads to an inability to respond to new environments and results in poorer balance. For example, if a stray rock has made its way onto the sidewalk, your gripping toes may not perceive that information and send it on to your brain, meaning that you're more likely to stumble because of it. If you have stiff toes, as many goldeners do, you're likely reinforcing that habit while you're exercising—even though you're exercising to try to make your body healthier! When we use these coping mechanisms over a long period of time, it's common to end up with toes that can't stop contracting and hip musculature that has never contracted. Stable balancing requires accessing the 360° of thigh muscles that do a better job than your clenching toes ever could. Watch for clenching toes during balance exercises and if you experience any of the common "fear of falling" reflexes, simply relax those muscles. You may have to relax gripping toes or clenched shoulders fifty times in a one-minute Pelvic List, but the more you recognize your unhelpful behavior, the faster you can change it.

CHAPTER 5

REACHING, CARRYING, LIFTING, AND OTHER FUNCTIONAL MOVEMENTS

Walking is one of the most important movements we do. Alongside walking, though, are other functional whole-body motions we can call on each day: getting up, getting down, carrying, lifting, reaching, taking the stairs, and touching your toes. These activities open up not only our knees, hips, and shoulders, but also the experiences available to you.

GETTING DOWN AND BACK UP AGAIN

The ability to comfortably transition between the ground or chair and standing is very under-rated. I can tell you from my experience working with many folks that it's sorely missed once it's gone. But here's the silver lining: it's not really gone—you're just out of practice, maybe by a handful of decades.

As simple as it seems, getting down and back up again requires joint mobility and enough muscular strength to lift our body away from the ground. We're full-grown humans! We're heavy!

Many goldeners find getting down to the ground and back up again daunting, so if you're one of them, rest assured you're in good company. In fact, many people of varying ages have lost the ability to rise from the floor with comfort. Our beds, couches, and chairs, as comfortable as they are, *prevent* us from making it down to the floor. And so we must slowly start using our body in the ranges of motion that have been stifled by use of furniture, until we redevelop enough strength in our legs, hips, and arms to carry us more easily.

If you're not regularly getting down to the floor, strengthening the muscles for this skill can start at chair level.

CHAIR SQUAT

You're already getting up multiple times a day—from your favorite chair, out of your car, and off the toilet. How you get up, though, dictates which muscles you're strengthening and

 Lora Says

I currently teach these exercises in a group class format. Part of my teaching strategy includes full disclosure of my continuing problems and spectacular victories. Students see me walking around town and will correct any errors they spot. It seems to me that if they see the errors in me they'll be more aware of them in themselves. I was at a concert where one of our students came up to me at the intermission and said, "I saw you use your arms to help you stand. Is that the best you can do tonight?" The "standing" reminder pleased me because we're making an impact on others and getting coaching ourselves.

which you're not. Common strategies for getting up without using much strength:

- Use momentum (giving it the ol' heave ho!).
- Push down with your arms.
- Pull yourself up with your arms.
- Shift your weight forward to use the muscles on the front of your thighs.

Try getting up and down a few times to see if you're currently using any of these methods and note which ones.

Strategies to help you start using more muscle:

- Decrease momentum (raise yourself slowly).
- Shift your weight back as you stand (pressing with your heels, NOT your toes).
- Lean forward with your chest and reach forward with your arms.
- Keep your knees in line with your hips (don't let them drop in toward each other).

The best way to incorporate these new getting-up techniques is to practice them first as an exercise.

Tip from the Goldeners

If you're not able to rise from the chair without lots of momentum, or if standing up with this form causes any pain, stack towels or place a book or yoga block on the seat to give yourself a little lift. As you get stronger, you can decrease the height of your bolster.

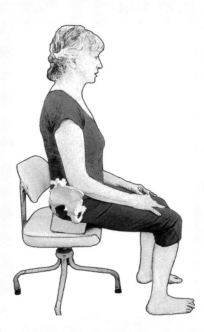

 Lora Says

When I first tried the standing exercise I saw that both my knees were attempting to knock together. By raising the height of the seat with two yoga blocks, I could stay aligned as I lifted or lowered myself. One day later I used only one block and in two more days I didn't need a prop at all. It was the fastest "fix" I've made and a very satisfying one, as I'd not even noticed the knee-knocking propensity before.

Start by sitting on a flat, hard chair (i.e., a kitchen chair). Scoot forward toward the front edge of the chair, tipping the top of your pelvis forward.

Adjust your feet so that your ankles stack directly below your knees.

Reaching your arms and leaning your torso forward, shift your weight back into your heels as you stand up, then rise, and then lower yourself slowly.

Once you start paying attention, you'll find that we lift and lower ourselves many times during the day. Exercises are an excellent place to train, but the next step is to make mindful form part of your life—whenever you stand up from or sit down on a flat chair, or sit down on and rise up from the toilet. All of the people I've worked with have found it advantageous to make every lift and lower a strength-builder.

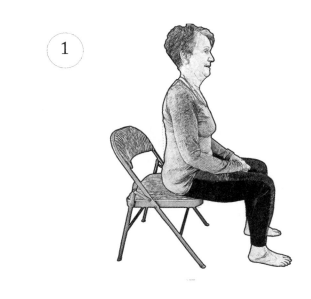

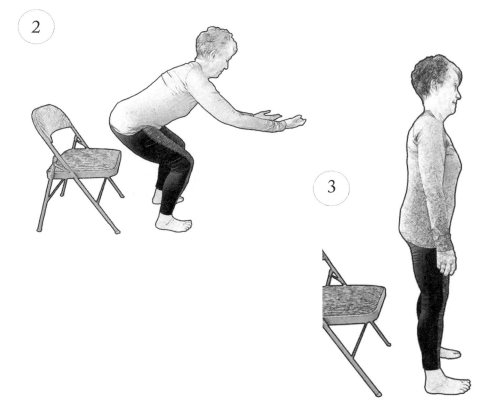

Cozy Chairs

Many of the chairs in our homes are cozy—puffy, stuffed, pillowed—and easy to sink into. They're the "dessert" version of furniture in that while they make us feel good, they're not always providing the best "movement nutrients."

Getting up and down from these chairs can be tricky because they don't often allow a body alignment that's conducive to using your muscles. If you're interested in strengthening your body, throughout the day opt for firmer chairs that require you to work your body more on the up, down, and lounge portions of sitting, and save the cushioned-up version of sitting for those times when you want to indulge.

TRAINING YOUR GET UP/GET DOWN MUSCLES

If you regularly attend an exercise class that includes floor work—like yoga or Pilates—you may already be able to get down to and up from the floor with ease. If this is you, start paying attention to how you're getting up. Check to see which leg and/or arm you depend on most. These are likely your stronger limbs. See if you can switch your lead leg and arm to more evenly condition your body.

Your floor is the best piece of exercise equipment you may not be using. Here are a few routines to try. Pick one each day and note how you do.

- Get up and down from the floor ten times in a row.
- Start seated on the ground and rise six times, each time choosing an alternating lead hand and foot.
- Start lying down on the floor and rising from your back three times and then from your abdomen three times.

CARRYING, LIFTING, AND REACHING

Just like the furniture in our homes makes it convenient to not use the muscles and joints of the lower body, other aspects of how we've arranged our homes have made it convenient to not have to use our arms much. This isn't only true of a golden-er's home—it's true of most homes in our culture.

For example, I grew up in a house with a kitchen organized in a way that ensured the things I needed to cook with were easy to access. Not only easier to find, but easier to reach.

"Easier to reach" is another way of saying "takes less movement." And so, to get your body moving more, you might consider rearranging your kitchen so that it takes more movement.

I don't mean you need to mix everything up so every meal requires many extra steps searching in vain for the item you can no longer find—just that you can arrange it so your day-to-day life requires that you reach up a little higher more often than you currently do, or squat or bend down a little lower Here are some suggestions to get you started:

- Place your tea or coffee filters on the top shelf.
- Put the mugs way down low.
- Put your plates at the back of a cupboard.
- Organize your refrigerator so that your most-used ingredients are in the most difficult-to-reach spot.

The last time I had dinner at my father's house, I went looking for a glass of wine, only to find he had taken my advice and was now storing the wine under the sink. "I get more shoulder and hip movement that way!" he said. (I don't know if I mentioned it yet, but my love of movement actually comes from my dad, who took me—forced me, really—on countless daily walks.)

CARRYING

Many people find that their back or shoulders hurt when they're carrying something. In the same way you can make over how you stand for better muscle recruitment, you can make over the way you're positioned when you carry to better use your legs, torso, and upper body.

Assume the position!

- Straight feet
- Weight back in heels
- Weight centered between your right and left legs
- Center your pelvis
- Center your ribcage

Using your arms to reach, hold, and carry requires a lot of shoulder strength and mobility—and shoulder strength and mobility require, you guessed it, a lot of arm movement. Carrying things requires that your arms and trunk muscles work well together, and these muscles depend on a stable torso. As you work to keep your ribcage down while walking and standing, you might find you feel very hunched over.

That's because one of the ways we mask the excessive curvature in the upper back is by lifting the chest (which is really the ribcage) up and out to make it look like we're standing up straight. While our heads are lifted and now stacked over our hips, the excessive curvature in our spine remains (and now we've also compressed our low back excessively). Here are some exercises to improve your shoulder and upper-spine mobility (letting you keep your ribs down and your head up) and your upper body strength.

RAMP YOUR HEAD

This postural adjustment is so important and effective, I'm including it twice. The human head is heavy. If you couple the weight of your head with the weakness of your upper body and a lot of computer and book-reading time, the result is a head out in front of the rest of the body. The other adjustments you're making to how much you move and how your body is positioned will help to improve this situation, but you need to be working on the alignment of your upper body as well. As often as you can—while walking, waiting in line, sitting at the computer, or driving in your car—slide your chin back while lengthening the back of your neck. This not only changes the placement of your head, it gets you using the muscles that are there to support your head.

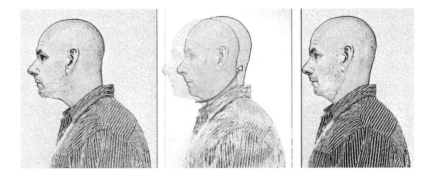

Swallowing Is Movement Too

Difficulty swallowing and choking while eating are prevalent issues in goldener populations—a phenomenon often chalked up to general weakness of all the muscles, including those in the throat. While this could be a contributing factor, the angles food has to move through to get from mouth to stomach can also impact the ease with which it's swallowed.

We think of food just having to move down into our stomachs, but in fact there are two stages of movement for food being swallowed: horizontal (from the front of your mouth to the back of the throat) and then vertical (down through your throat).

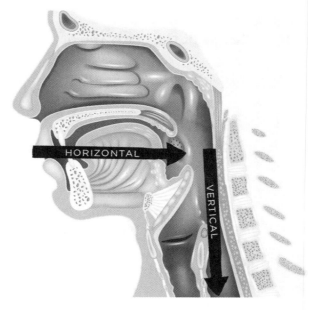

If your head is often out in front of you, a position that not only slightly lifts your chin (think how your head would be positioned while looking through a lower bifocal lens) but also places your throat on a diagonal, your position alone makes the movement of food harder. Next time you eat, remember that your head position is directly related to throat position and can be affecting the space and work necessary to get food down safely. Yes, cut and chew your food well, but also, mind your posture when you're eating and see if you notice a difference!

FLOOR ANGELS

Begin by reclining on a bolster or stacked pillows so that your ribcage can lower toward the floor. Stretch your legs out straight.

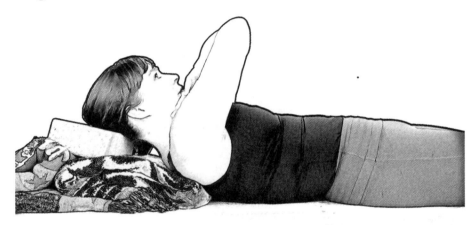

Reach your arms out to the sides, keeping your palms facing up and your elbows rotating up in the direction of the ceiling. Lower your arms and the backs of your hands toward the floor, keeping your elbows slightly bent. Once you've opened your arms as far as they can go, slowly move them up toward your head—like you're making snow angels. Try some however you can, and then try some only going as far as you can keeping your thumbs on the floor.

Once you've done this for a while, try a few times monitoring your ribcage position—making sure that your ribs are staying down and not raising up as your arms move overhead.

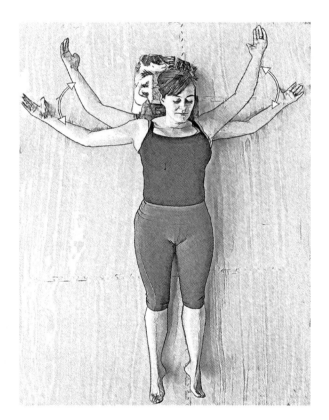

THORACIC STRETCH

Stand facing a wall, countertop, or back of a chair (start higher and work your way down over time). Placing both hands on the wall (or other support), slowly back up until your arms are fully outstretched, lowering your chest through your arms. If you can, straighten your legs and shift your weight back toward your heels so you can easily wiggle your toes. Allow your neck to relax and your head to drop.

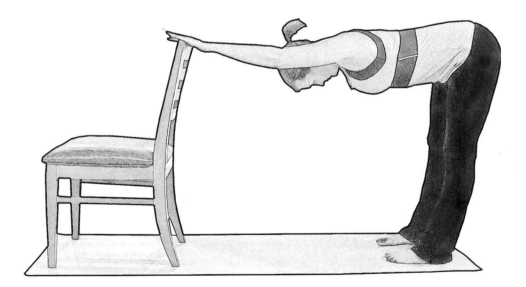

DOORWAY REACH

Reach your arms up until you can touch the wall above the doorway, and then lower your ribcage down as much as you can. If you can't do both arms at once, do one arm at a time walking your fingers up the wall to the right of a doorway, as far as you can. Lowering your ribs will intensify the motion in your arms and shoulders. Repeat both sides.

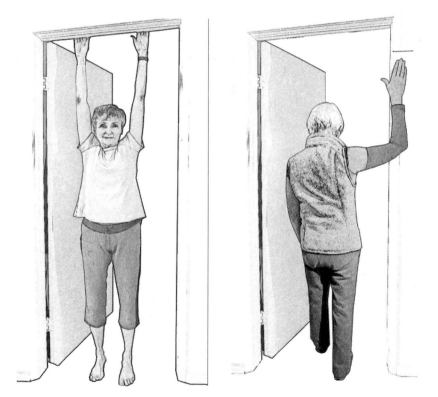

Check the position of your elbows. Do they always point outward? Try a few with your elbows pointing straight ahead and see how this movement changes the stretch in the arms, shoulders, and torso.

If you're getting up and moving more throughout the day, you'll find yourself walking through doorways more often. Each time you do is a chance to spend ten to fifteen seconds moving your arms and shoulders in new ways and fitting more movement into your day!

STRENGTHEN THE MUSCLES BETWEEN YOUR RIBS

Breath can move in and out of your body in many ways, and one of those ways requires the movement of your ribs. This movement keeps the muscles in your ribcage strong, which can come in handy when you need to do things like cough—a movement essential to a well-functioning breathing system. To mobilize and strengthen this area, try the following exercise.

Seated or standing in the aligned position, firmly tie an elastic resistance band or pair of pantyhose or tights around your ribcage, just beneath your chest muscles or breasts (at the height of a bra strap or heart-rate monitor). If you don't have anything, place your hands on your hips then slide them up until they're on the sides of your ribcage, and lightly press as if to hold the ribcage narrow.

Inhale slowly, trying to stretch the band by expanding the ribcage. If you don't feel the band's tension increase at the end of your inhale, re-tie the band a little more snugly and try it again.

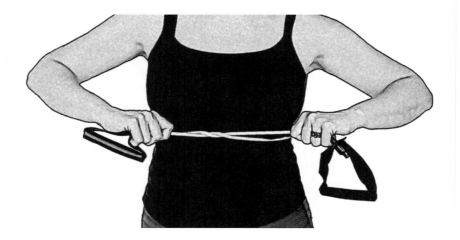

Exhale, being aware of how your ribcage can pull away from the ring of elastic and closer to an imaginary vertical pole running up through the center of your body. Repeat, using each exhale to bring the ribs inward.

Now instead of exhaling, try a slow cough in the same position, bringing the ribs inward.

You should find (feel!) that breathing, especially the exhale, engages the muscles between the ribs and throughout the abdomen. You can use the elastic to teach you how to find and use these muscles, but once you've got the motor skill, you can do this exercise without the tactile assistance of the band.

TAKING THE STAIRS WITH EASE

Whether there are two to three steps up to your house or an entire flight to your second story, steps are a part of everyday life for most of us. Out of all the "real life" movements people do, I hear the most complaints about knees on the stairs. The size and shape of steps are fixed, and don't usually match well to the stride

Joyce Says

I began walking to do all my errands each day a few years ago, after I moved to where I had a three- to four-mile radius from my house to the city business areas. The challenge for me was to find how I could carry my bags and knapsack and maintain my balance, and balance the weight on my body. My preferred method of carrying bags of groceries, bottles of water, and some cartons and bags with fragile or delicate contents soon became apparent to me. The heavier bottles of water were carried most easily balanced on my horizontal forearm and hugged against my torso or hoisted up to my shoulder, where their weight was easy to hold and balance. The knapsack rode easily on my back and could be loaded with contents that did not jab into me as I walked. The more fragile bags of food were carried either hugged lightly next to my body or carried in my hands.

I enjoy the challenge of accommodating the varying loads to my body and the experience of carrying everything I buy home with me. At first I puffed when under a heavy load, but gradually my strength grew, and I now accomplish it all without strain and with a lot of enjoyment and feeling of accomplishment. Whole-body movement is a possible lifestyle in urban areas—just saying!

length we would choose to take naturally were we on a hill. Steps work better for people with certain limb lengths and are much harder to accommodate for people with other limb lengths.

While there's not much we can do about the fixed shape and size of a step, we can change the shape of our body as we take the stairs—which often alleviates pain and can improve strength at the same time.

Tip 1: Keep your torso upright. One of the reasons we lean forward is to use momentum instead of leg muscle. Keeping your torso vertical will make your legs work more, which will make them stronger and make you more capable of taking the stairs.

Tip 2: Check your knees. As you're stepping up, look down at your stepping-up leg's knee. Does it collapse inward or outward as you step up or down? Use the muscles in your hip to hold your knee in the same plane as your ankle—adjust your knee inward or outward to get it centered. This will keep you from using the ligaments of the knee and increase the amount of muscle you're using.

Tip 3: Use your calves more! As you walk upstairs, don't just use the front leg to pull you up—push off with the foot on your back leg as well. This not only reduces the load to the knee, it keeps your calf strength up. As you go down stairs, you may notice that you land on the lower step with your toes pointed. Instead of quickly crashing from your toes to your heel, slow

Joan Says

We live on a ten-acre ranch on the side of a mountain in a forest of coastal oaks and black walnut trees. While developing the land to build our home, in my early sixties, I would carry a twenty- to twenty-five-pound sprayer backpack for weed abatement. Being on a mountain, some of the hillsides are very steep and slippery, making it difficult for me to keep my balance and footing, especially with weight on my back. So, we put in some three hundred individual wooden steps in the very steep areas around the perimeter to facilitate this annual task. I no longer carry the spray backpack; however, I continue to alternate hiking our trail system with going up and down the steps to work my quads, hamstrings, balance, and endurance.

down and let your calf muscles control your descent. This, too, uses the muscles around the knees less and your calves more!

I suggest practicing each of these tips as separate exercises, where you're paying attention to form. Then, when you take the stairs, this improved form will come naturally to you!

 ## Shelah Says

I am one lucky person! For thirty-five years I have lived in the same second-floor apartment that gives me lower-body strengthening every day without any extra time or planning. Then, fifteen years ago, my studio moved to the third floor. More "no extra time or planning" movement strengthening.

I would be remiss not to mention that at times the stairs have been a challenge, especially when my back was injured. In that case it was slow and steady, with gratitude for the sturdy railings.

Heavily loaded bags can also be a problem. I leave the bag at the bottom of the stairs and carry up the contents in manageable loads. If all else fails I ask for help from my eldest son, who lives with me, or from understanding neighbors.

For me the answer to staying mobile is lifestyle, making "practice" part of my daily routine.

The Importance of Reaching Your Toes

The shoes you choose to wear could be increasing your risk of falling. In one study researchers found that the footwear most often worn at the time of a fall-related hip fracture were shoes that didn't attach properly to the foot, like slippers or slip-ons (Sherrington and Menz 2003). Slip-on footwear often appeals to goldeners because it takes less effort (read: I don't have to bend over) to get them on.

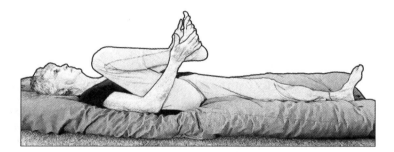

If you're having trouble reaching down to put on or tie up footwear, try this movement. Lie on your back (doing this each morning before you get out of bed is a great idea) and, maintaining a relaxed breath, bring one knee toward your chest.

Can you reach your foot with one hand? Can you grab that foot with both hands at the same time? Try the other side. Work up to being able to hold each foot in both hands in this position for one minute.

Having enough mobility to reach our feet is crucial. This not only prevents the progression to slide-on-only footwear, but also enables other aspects of foot care, like toenail maintenance, splinter removal, and callus care—all extremely important for all of us, including goldeners!

SQUAT TO POT

There's a form to walking and there's a form to taking the stairs and yes, there's a form to toileting as well!

Relatively speaking, toilets are a recent invention. Until we started using them exclusively, humans squatted to eliminate. As inconvenient as that may seem to our joints that have never had to do this motion, squatting, it turns out, is very convenient for our internal pipes and tubes involved in toileting.

Straining to toilet is often a direct result of poor alignment of our "eliminating tube" (the descending colon)—so much so

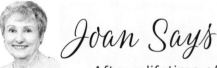

Joan Says

After a lifetime of constipation and difficulty eliminating, I am now, after my movement program—which includes squatting to toilet using a Squatty Potty—symptom free. Elimination is regular and without any effort. Accomplishing this health benefit is huge. In addition, I have strength in my hips, knees, and ankles that I didn't have before. My ankles don't "give way" suddenly when I'm walking as they did before I began moving differently and more, including squatting to toilet.

that squatting protocols have been added in physical therapy treatments of the pelvic floor and digestive system.

One way to get into a toileting alignment with ease is to use a squat platform—a low-profile stool that wraps around the front of your toilet, gently lifting your knees into the squatting position while sitting on the toilet. For many, this simple adjustment not only gets them moving their knees and hips more, but allows for an easier movement—if you catch my drift.

Goldeners and the Pelvic Floor

Many goldeners experience pelvic floor issues, from incontinence to pelvic organ prolapse to prostate problems. Pelvic floor disorders tend to be thought of as a "goldener" issue, but it's really a phenomenon increasing across many demographics. As with many other diseases and ailments, I've found pelvic floor disorders to often be the symptom of a mostly sedentary lifestyle—correctable through more mindful movement practices (moving more), better standing and sitting alignment, and a change in habits that cause pressure on pelvic organs and the pelvic floor. If you're experiencing any kind of pelvic floor disorder, you might notice that some of the exercises and adjustments in this book decrease the symptoms of things like incontinence, pressure, and pain. The issue is much too large to address comprehensively in this book, but there are many other resources available, including the additional exercises used by these goldeners to improve their prolapse symptoms. Find them in the Appendix, page 237.

CHAPTER 6

FIT TO DRIVE

Not using your car because you'd rather walk to the post office or grocery store is great, but maintaining the physical ability to drive can be a major factor in your independence and thus your happiness. The physical ability to drive has to do not only with our eyes and ears; we also need motor skills, joint mobility, strength, and fast reaction time in order to drive safely. These are things you can work to improve by, you guessed it, moving more.

While there have been no specific studies that link musculoskeletal health to accidents, the lack of mobility commonly associated with aging is definitely a risk factor for accidents, and something doctors screen for when they're deciding whether or not to revoke a goldener's driving privileges (American Geriatrics Society and Pomidor 2016).

Though driving is a fairly sedentary activity, there are definitely motions you need to be able to execute in order to drive safely. For example, you need to be able to rotate your neck and trunk to look behind you when you're backing up or changing lanes. You need shoulder, elbow, and hand mobility for rapid handling of the steering wheel when you're making sharp turns. You need ankle mobility and control to effectively depress the gas, brake, and clutch pedals. And finally, you need general foot health—especially the foot's sensory and motor nerves, to ensure you're using the correct pedal.

I live in a small city filled with goldeners—40 percent of the population is over sixty-five—and it is not uncommon to see the side of a building smashed in by a car. In my first two years here, I saw the side of a building or a guard pole smashed by cars on five separate occasions. Because it's a "small town," I was able to gather that, most frequently, these accidents were not the result of the driver mixing up, cognitively, the brake pedal for the gas pedal—they mistakenly sensed they had moved their foot over when they hadn't. The brain's ability to know where the foot is in space requires our proprioceptive system (your ability to sense where your body is in space) to be well-functioning, and the foot's intrinsic muscles and nerves, as well as the muscles and nerves that connect to it, to be healthy.

DRIVING-SPECIFIC MOVEMENTS

Everyone wants to stay in shape. You can think of driving as a sport, where there are specific movements to master, and train just as an athlete would. Step one is to evaluate how well you're currently executing the motions necessary for driving. Step two is to start using them more frequently. Below is a list of mobility tests and correctives to keep your body sound for many functional tasks, including driving.

THE SIT AND TWIST TEST

Sit in a chair with both feet on the ground, pelvis sitting evenly on the seat, and hands resting on your lap. Rotate your ribcage without letting either hip lift off the chair. Can you see behind you yet? Keeping your ribcage rotated, try also rotating your head to continue the twisting motion. How about now? Are you able to rotate your upper body enough to see behind you, or do you have to lift one side of your pelvis and use your arms to compensate for too-tight muscles?

There's nothing much in our regular daily life that requires we use the twisting action of our waist and so, because we rarely do it, we lose the ability. To restore lost motion, add these exercises to your daily routine.

THE BACKING UP TWIST

Aligning your pelvis and rib cage before you twist can help you better target the muscles of the waist. Adjust your pelvis so it's not overly tucked or overly tipped forward (see Center Your Pelvis, pages 90–91) and lower the bottom front of the ribcage so it stacks over the front of the pelvis. Without lifting your ribcage or tucking or untucking your pelvis, turn to the right without straining, and hold 20–30 seconds. Repeat on the left.

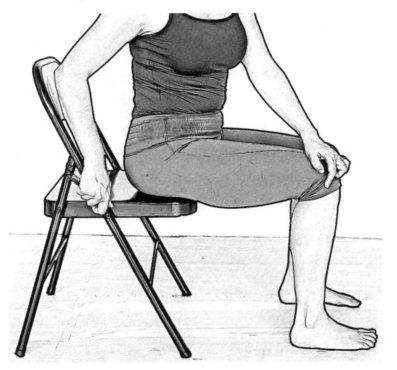

BOLSTERED FLOOR TWIST

Place a pillow or two under your head and shoulders to bring the bottom of your ribcage to the ground. Stretch your legs out in front of you, and reach your arms out to the sides to make a T (this will help you keep your upper body stationary as you rotate your lower half).

Scoot your pelvis an inch or two to the right, bring your right knee up so that it stacks over your hip, then rotate your

Joan Says

Before I started with Katy, I was finding it more and more difficult to turn my head and ribs without lifting my opposite hip to look behind me and now, thanks to the correctives, I can turn and keep my hips squarely in the seat. Additionally, I have seen changes in my hyperkyphosis (chin jutting forward and up) by ramping my head as I drive to get the back of my head against the headrest. When I started, the back of my head was probably four inches away from the head rest. Now, without effort (other than being aware of what I am doing) I can rest the back of my head against the head rest and keep my eyes looking straight ahead on the road.

pelvis to lower that knee across the body, stopping as soon as your ribs start to twist away from the ground.

Twist only as far as you can without taking the ribs with you—you don't want to force this move.

If you find that your pelvis barely moves and your knee is nowhere near the floor, that's fine—just **stack pillows so that the knee crossing over can rest on them.**

Repeat on the other side.

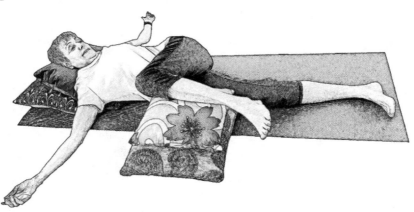

Lora Says

Regular twisting has eliminated my creaky neck syndrome (a term I coined myself!). The best part is that I have free neck movement to look behind me before lane changes, which has occasionally saved me from a world of hurt.

THE ANKLE MOBILITY TEST

Get into a lunge position on the ground, with your front foot's big toe four inches (three inches if you are under 5'2") from the wall. Without lifting your front heel from the ground,

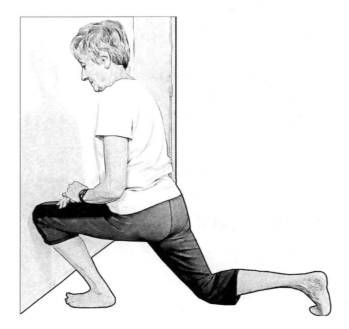

can you touch your knee to the wall? If not, then your ankle's range of motion is limited, which could affect your ability to raise your foot easily off the gas or brake pedal. (While those of us driving automatic cars only have one "pedal" foot, still take this test and do the correctives with both feet!)

To improve your ankle's range of motion, revisit the calf-stretching exercises on pages 60 to 63. It turns out that keeping your ankles fit for driving also keeps them fit for walking and vice versa. The takeaway here is all mobility goes hand-in-hand! And speaking of hands…

THE HAND-SHOULDER MOBILITY TEST

Tight hands can be weak hands and can also be connected to stiff shoulders. Having the ability to react quickly and accurately with your hands, arms, and shoulders is important for safe driving. Fortunately, you can improve your hands and shoulders at the same time with this exercise.

Get down on your hands and knees (**or, if that's not a feasible position for you right now, stand with your arms reaching forward to a wall**) and arrange your hands so that the middle finger on each hand is pointing straight forward (or straight up, if you're standing at a wall). (See images top of page 146.)

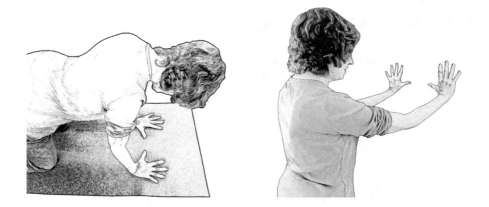

Thumb/shoulder assessment: Move your thumbs away from your fingers until they point directly toward each other, i.e., perpendicular to the middle fingers.

Once you've spread your thumbs out, check in with your shoulders: Are your elbows turning to point outward?

Can you keep your fingers and thumbs spread while pulling your elbows inward, or does pulling your elbows require your thumbs to move toward your other fingers? (Top images on opposite page.)

Hand assessment: Are your hands flat and relaxed on the floor or are some of your finger joints bending? (Bottom images on opposite page.)

YES

*ELBOWS PULLED TOWARD
EACH OTHER*

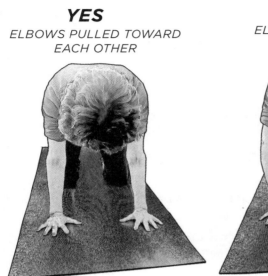

NO

*ELBOWS POINTING
OUTWARD*

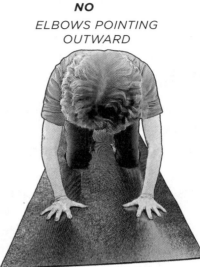

YES

FINGER JOINTS EXTENDING

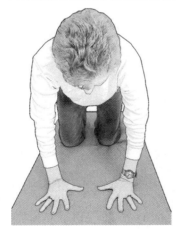

NO

SOME FINGER JOINTS BENT

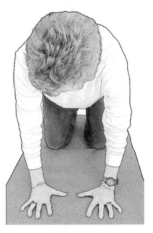

If your thumbs move when your arms do, or if your fingers can't straighten all the way, it's time for some exercises that help decrease tension in the tissues between the wrist, elbow, and shoulder.

HANDS ON THE FLOOR (OR WALL)

This isn't only a test—getting down on to your hands and knees to spread your fingers (or placing your hands flat on a wall in front of you) daily will help you improve the motion in these areas. Lining up your elbows so that the pointy part of your elbow points opposite to your middle fingers will work on your shoulders too. And speaking of elbows...

ELBOW TOUCH

With your arms out in front of your body, elbows bent at 90° and palms facing you, bring your elbows together until they touch. (See image top of next page.)

Keeping the elbows together, move your wrists away from each other. Once you can do this with greater ease, start doing it while also making sure your shoulder blades stay down (keep shoulders from hiking up toward your ears).

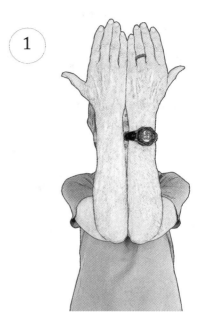

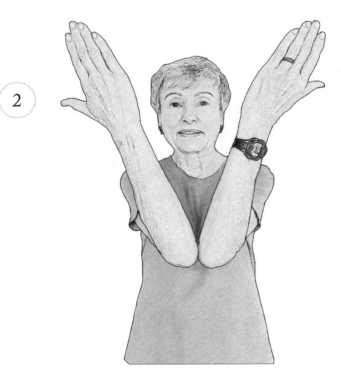

FINGER STRETCHES

Place one hand out in front like you're signing STOP. Keeping that elbow bent and pointed to the ground, pull each finger back one at a time with your other hand until you feel a stretch. Pay close attention to the finger you are stretching to make sure none of its three joints are bending.

YES   **NO** (FINGER JOINTS BENT)

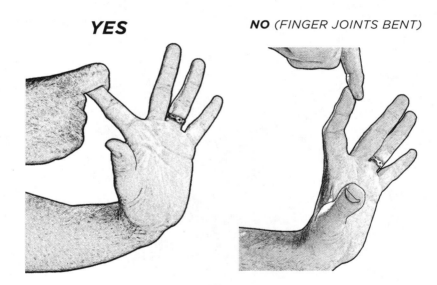

THE RAPID-PACE WALKING TEST

This is an objective test of functional lower-body strength, balance, and agility used by the American Geriatrics Society to determine if a goldener driver is at-risk.

Set up a ten-foot path on the floor, marked with masking tape, and get a stopwatch (or a friend who'll time you with the second hand).

Start your stopwatch, then walk to the end of the path, turn, and walk back as quickly as possible. If it takes you longer than nine seconds, your score is associated with an increased risk of an at-fault motor accident.

In addition to regularly working through the exercises in this book and increasing the amount of walking you're doing on a daily basis, consider adding a little "faster than regular" walking in areas safe from debris or trip hazards. Your hallway could be a dedicated safe sprinting zone. Every time you walk down it, kick up your speed a bit to train your go-fast muscles! Check back with this assessment every month or so and see if your time improves.

THE GET UP AND GO TEST

In the Get Up and Go Test (American Geriatrics Society and Pomidor 2016, 44), you begin by sitting in a straight-backed chair. Then you have to:

- rise from the chair,

- stand still momentarily,

- walk a short distance (around ten feet or three meters),

- turn around,

- walk back to the chair,

- turn around,

- and sit down again.

Those taking the test are rated on their stability and likelihood of falling. It's not every day you practice getting up, walking, and turning. Adding these moves to your life can improve how you do them, and the exercises in this book can make these easier for you—especially those parts used in the "getting down and getting back up again" section beginning on page 108.

DRIVING TEST CHEAT SHEET

We all had to take a test to get our driver's license and many, eventually, have to take a test to be able to *keep* it. In addition to cognition and vision exams, being considered fit to drive requires that you pass

> "Studying for tests can improve results, so why not "study" by keeping your body strong and supple enough to drive safely?

mobility and motor skill tests administered by a doctor. Studying for tests can improve results, so why not "study" by keeping your body strong and supple enough to drive safely? Here are some of the tests as described in the *Clinician's Guide to Assessing*

Driving Requires Healthy Feet!

Remember the toe spreading we did on page 36, and the toe-lifting on page 42? Those fine-motor foot skills are indicators of more than you might think. Intrinsic foot-muscle atrophy—that is, the weakness of the muscles that reside entirely within the foot—can be an early indicator of a loss of nerve health in the lower leg (Greenman et al. 2005). Do your "toe exercises" regularly to strengthen the muscles and improve the health of the nerves (Balducci et al. 2006)! See, even driving requires healthy feet! See chapter 1 for toe exercises.

and Counseling Older Drivers, 3rd Edition. (American Geriatrics Society and Pomidor 2016). Alongside each test, I'll note which exercises can improve your results.

MOVEMENT TEST	THE PHYSICIAN SAYS	EXERCISES TO "STUDY"
Neck rotation	"Look over your shoulder like you're backing up and parking. Now do the same thing for the other side."	· **Seated and Supported Spinal Twist** · **Head Ramping**
Shoulder and elbow flexion	"Pretend you're holding a steering wheel. Now pretend to make a wide right turn, then a wide left turn."	· **Elbow Touch** · **Floor Angels** · **Doorway Reach**
Finger curl	"Make a fist with both of your hands."	· **Finger Stretches**
Ankle plantar flexion	"Pretend you're stepping on the gas pedal. Now do the same for the other foot."	· **All Foot Exercises**
Ankle dorsiflexion	"Point your toes toward your body."	· **Calf Stretch 1** · **Calf Stretch 2**

(AMERICAN GERIATRICS SOCIETY AND POMIDOR 2016, 45)

Less driving-specific movement tests include general mobility tests. Below are some of the general movements that may be tested and the exercises to help you strengthen and mobilize these areas:

MOVEMENT TEST	EXERCISES TO "STUDY"
Shoulders: reaching out, across, and behind you	· **Floor Angels** · **Doorway Reach**
Wrist flexion and extension	· **Hand Stretches**
Hand-grip strength	· **Hand Stretches**
Hip flexion and extension	· **Walking** · **Top of the Foot Stretch**
Ankle dorsiflexion and plantar flexion	· **Calf Stretch 1 and 2** · **Foot Exercises**

CHAPTER 7
MOVEMENT IS PART OF LIFE

We went back and forth over the name of this book. *Aging* is a term often applied to older generations, but the fact of the matter is we're *all* aging, from the day we're born. Aging is an inevitable part of life, and it doesn't indicate anything other than the fact that our time and experience are constantly accumulating—which is truly a gift.

Dynamic aging, though—that is something else entirely. Dynamic aging requires movement. Dynamic aging is the acquisition of time and experience alongside the acquisition of physical skill. While we're all aging, we're not all aging dynamically, for this requires that we move.

Our tissues do change with age, but they also change through lack of movement. When you couple older tissues with a longer habit of not moving much (which we all have; it's very easy to get by in our culture with very little movement), you wind up with a body that feels unable to go out and gather the experiences of life you desire.

Our culture's perspective is that this decline in movement is related to aging, but I want to stress again that our culture is sedentary. All of us in our culture have spent the bulk of our lives unmoving, and so the transformative effects of movement are rarely considered as being integral to all aspects of life, including aging.

That all said, most scientists and medical professionals will tell you that you need to start exercising, because research shows just how protective of health this can be. However, exercise time is typically allotted to a tiny fraction of each day. If movement is hugely transformative, why not learn to put the movement, beyond exercise, back into each day?

We are used to thinking of exercise as something we do "outside" the obligations of our regular life. Thus our obligations keep us from moving abundantly through life because our families and jobs and community work and housework take our attention. Exercise is a great asset, but few have the luxury of bumping up their exercise time to three or four hours each day. You can, however, get your body moving closer to that amount by setting your life up in a way that requires more movement.

This book is full of exercises and even a workout routine at the end, but it's also full of ways to put more movement back into the daily tasks you're already doing. I've found this to be key to improved movement in all populations, from toddlers to competitive athletes to goldeners to new mothers fresh from birthing their children.

Lora Says

I've found some of my most powerful routine movement comes from aligning my beliefs with my activities.

I carry my wet wash out to hang in the sun. If it's cold enough for my heat to be on, I hang the laundry on racks inside, which provides moisture for the heated air.

I have seven rain barrels and get the whole-body challenge of distributing water where it's most needed.

I have buckets in my shower to catch the cold water that precedes my luxurious warm shower. The cold water rinses dirty dishes. All the water I use in food prep, which has vitamins in it, gets carried to plantings in special need in my half-acre yard.

Composting adds enormously to amassing ten thousand steps per day. And don't cross out composting just because you have clay soil with no worms. Shelah's compost provides me with worms, and I give them material for their worm projects.

These ways of exercising provide physical endorphins, defined shoulder muscles (for the first time in my life), stronger joints and muscles, and the satisfaction that I'm doing a good job as present caretaker of my land—a cause I am most passionate about.

Our bodies require movement—a lot of it—to operate fully. This is the reason exercise is almost always listed as beneficial for health issues. And it's not only the muscles and joints that movement protects. A lack of exercise can affect the health of your eyes (and thus vision [Zheng et al. 2015]), brain (cognition and memory; see sidebar below), and digestion (De Schryver et al. 2005); it can negatively impact your energy levels, lipid panel results, and simply how good you feel each day. And a lack of exercise could be causing your cells to *age*

Exercise and Alzheimer's Disease

The details of how exercise helps prevent diseases and their progress is not always understood. But in one study, healthy, cognitively intact participants with a higher genetic risk for Alzheimer's disease were able to maintain hippocampal volume (the area of the brain known to shrink with Alzheimer's) with physical activity compared to those with low amounts of physical activity. (Smith et al. 2014) Geriatrician Katalin Koller, M.D. says, "When I talk with my patients, it is very important to discuss optimization of physical activity, contingent on their current ability and any personal limitations. I recommend physical activity not only because of the protective cognitive benefits, but for mental health and overall personal well-being."

faster. According to one researcher of the effect of diet and movement on aging:

> "Some of us believe that aging is just something that happens to all of us and it's just a predestined fate, and by the time I turn 65 or 70 or 80, I will have Alzheimer's disease and cardiovascular disease and osteoporosis," says Dr. LeBrasseur. "And this [study] clearly shows the importance of modifiable factors, so healthy diet, and even more so, just the importance of regular physical activity. So that doesn't mean that we need to be marathon runners, but we need to find ways to increase our habitual activity levels to stay healthy and prevent processes that drive aging and aging-related diseases." (Mayo Clinic 2016)

But how is it that we can age faster? As I said earlier in this chapter, we're all aging at the same rate. Or are we?

Each of your cells has a limited number of times it can divide; this is why our bodies don't last forever. The number of times your cells can divide is determined by the rate of loss of the protective caps (called telomeres; see sidebar page 163) of each chromosome

Telomeres

Telomeres are best thought of as the plastic cap on your shoelaces that prevent the laces unraveling. Once they are gone, the DNA is unstable, just like the thread of a lace without the cap, and it is too risky to allow the cell to continue to divide. Certain lifestyle factors like a poor diet, inflammation, and a lack of movement can accelerate cell divisions and the rate you're losing the telomeres on your chromosomes. What this means is that you—dear reader— have two ages. One age is determined by your birth- date (your chronological age) and the other is the age of your cells (your biological age). Your biological (cell) age depends on how fast you've prompted your cells to divide and how well your DNA is maintained through lifestyle- related factors.

at each cell division. Once a cell has stopped dividing, it becomes what is termed a "senescent" cell. Senescent cells are still active, but are associated with the production of inflammatory molecules and contribute to many age-related diseases.

The possible number of cell divisions we experience is not a fixed amount but rather a range that varies (adults range be- tween fifty to seventy divisions). Although we all accumulate days at the same rate, our cells are not all dividing at the same rate, and also the amount of telomere DNA lost at each cell division is not the same—which means two people of the same chronological age could have a different biological age, each having a different number of cellular divisions remaining before their cells become senescent.

Movement matters to your body on the cellular level. And so, instead of writing the typical book of "here are safe exercises for seniors," we want to say loud and clear that there are daily movements available—at every age—that focus on the dynamic part of aging. Movements that not only put movement back into your life, but also life into your cells. And in the end, this is the reason I've spent my life writing and teaching about why movement needs to play a large role in our life. It's not so that we can age dynamically, but so that we can *live* dynamically.

GET MOVING

ALL-DAY ALIGNMENT CHECKS

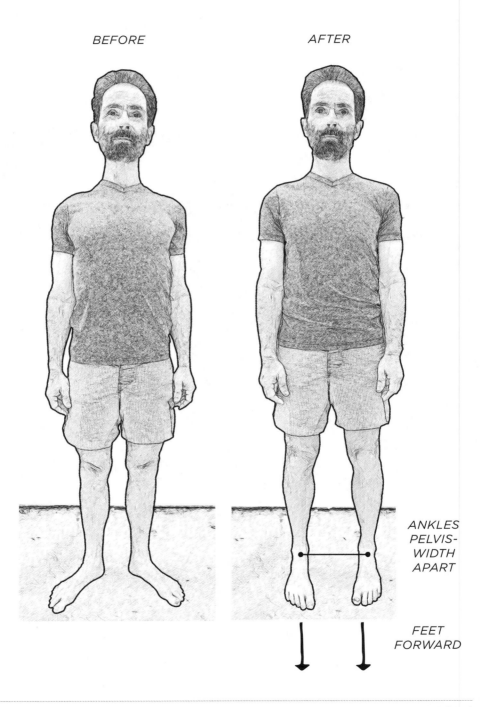

BEFORE

AFTER

ANKLES
PELVIS-
WIDTH
APART

FEET
FORWARD

DYNAMIC AGING

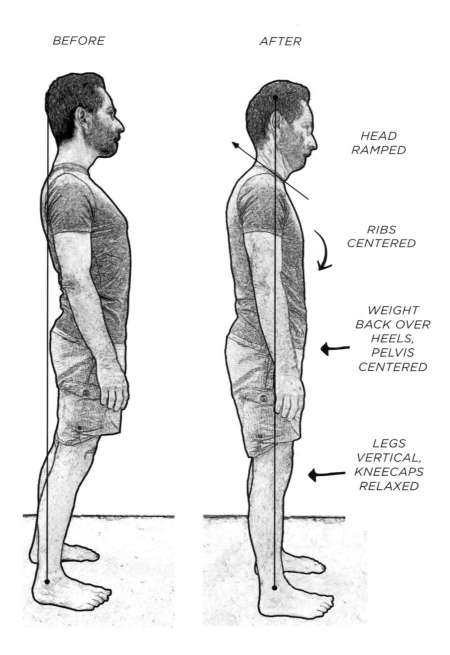

BEFORE

AFTER

HEAD
RAMPED

RIBS
CENTERED

WEIGHT
BACK OVER
HEELS,
PELVIS
CENTERED

LEGS
VERTICAL,
KNEECAPS
RELAXED

TIPS FOR MOVING MORE
IN DAILY LIFE

There are exercises to help you move better, and then there are small adjustments you can make to how you're living your life each day that will help you move more. Combining the two—an exercise practice with a move-through-your-life make-over—has brought about tremendous results for many. Here are some ways to get started.

CHANGE YOUR CLOSET

- Every morning you're putting on clothes and socks and shoes that affect how you move. When purchasing new clothes, check to see if your arms reach easily over head, or if a waistband pinches when you bend over (thus discouraging you from bending over!).

- As you dress, be aware of how you are moving. For example, can you balance on one foot to pull on your pants? You may need to lean against something to start; however, getting started is the key. Select shoes that allow your feet and ankles to move and strengthen fully.

Joan Says

I use my closet and getting dressed as an opportunity to integrate some of the correctives I have learned and to test my awareness. For example, I have taught myself to balance on one leg/foot when I am pulling on a pair of pants. I started by leaning against a wall—now I am able to do it freestanding. When I pull a shirt on over my head, I first drop my ribs and then check to see how well I can keep them down while reaching overhead. I have the most fun putting on my socks now that I wear toe-socks, which are shaped more like gloves than mittens, with a separate channel for each toe.

(sidebar cont'd next page)

(sidebar cont'd from previous page)

About two years ago, I noticed I could not maintain my balance for the time it took to stand and pull on my socks and shoes. So I started by leaning against a wall, pulling up one knee to my chest, then with sock in hand, reaching down to grab my foot. That took a while just to reach it. (Katy's suggested corrective on page 132 of lying on your back and pulling your knee in toward your chest to reach your foot is a great way to start stretching the necessary muscles.) Once I get ahold of my foot, I pull the sock on up to my instep. Then, still standing on one foot, I cross the sock foot over the knee of the standing foot and pretend I am going to sit in a chair, lowering my hips. Now using one or both hands, I get each toe into its separate channel. It has taken me two years to be able to do it pretty much freestanding—and it's been well worth the effort. The result has been a noticeable improvement in my overall balance. The other thing I have found helpful is to passively stretch my toes (when I am not on my feet) by wearing toe separators (like when you get a pedicure) or socks specially designed for toe separating (e.g., Foot Alignment Socks). I also actively stretch my toes (when standing or walking) by using an orthotic called Correct Toes that keeps the toes separated. I have seen a measurable improvement in the space between my toes, which also has helped my balance.

RETHINK YOUR FURNITURE

- Don't always sit in the same chair—mix it up between soft and hard, and with varying heights.

- Create an alternate work station, one that allows you to stand up or sit on a pillow on the floor to write letters or pay bills.

- If you're working on a computer, consider changing your setup—try putting the screen and/or keyboard at a different height from usual, or making the whole thing a standing work station.

- Leave a half foam roller wherever you stand for a few minutes at a time—where you do the dishes or brush your teeth.

- Create or buy a squat platform for use in your most-used bathroom.

- Sit on the floor instead of your couch or chair at least once a day.

GET YOUR KITCHEN MORE MOVEMENT-RICH

- Place your tea or coffee filters on the top shelf and the mugs way down low.

- Put your plates at the back of a cupboard and your napkins on top of the fridge.

- Organize your refrigerator so that your most-used ingredients are in the most difficult-to-reach spot.

- Cook with more old-fashioned implements—knead bread yourself, use a knife or moulé or potato masher instead of a food processor, use mortar and pestle instead of buying processed herbs.

 Lora Says

I've made a point to keep my home movement-friendly. I have a very large living room/dining room but have little furniture for it, and what I have is usually around the edges. A musician friend came in and excitedly cried, "It's alive, it's alive!" in reference to the slight echo of the room. My granddaughter came in shortly after and she and a friend immediately began dancing, which they kept up until they were exhausted and panting on the floor. All movement needs space, and apparently the more space available, the more the spirit can soar.

I've had many wonderful responses to the grand empty-ish room over the years, including more than fifty people dancing at my seventy-fifth birthday party, impromptu music sessions, and of course my own frequent use of the joy-inspiring space.

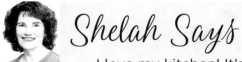

Shelah Says

I love my kitchen! It's my happy place. When we remodeled the kitchen in 1991, I got what I always wanted: lots of open counter space, two sinks, and lots of open shelves (because I'm one of those people who can't find it if I can't see it.)

Some of the open shelves are high, so I keep a stool handy and do a lot of reaching. Some of the cabinets are low, so I also do plenty of squatting and bending.

We didn't want to waste storage space on a dishwasher, and on a plant-based diet I don't eat much processed food, so I spend a lot of time washing dishes and chopping vegetables. I make sure I'm not standing with my hips against the counter with my weight forward (bad habit). I keep my weight back on my heels, and when I remember, I put a half dome under the counter so I can stretch my calves while I work. Or I do an alternating hip list, no equipment needed. I'm a messy cook, so I have to get down on my hands and knees frequently to mop up the floor.

But best of all, I recently got an electric pressure cooker that makes cooking super fast, so I can get OUT of the kitchen to go to class and move and walk more!

USE THE CAR LESS

- Walk to do errands.

- Walk to the grocery store a few times a week and carry home smaller amounts of groceries.

- If you need to drive, park a block or two away from where you're going.

NATURE

- Buy a few plants to spread throughout your home. Not only do you benefit from this tiny green space, you'll need to move more to tend to them.

- Take your book club or church group to the woods for a meeting instead of in a building.

- Swap a weekly neighborhood or treadmill walk for one on a path outside in a local park or wilderness area.

COMMUNITY

- Find a walking buddy or start a walking group.

- When you meet with your book club or church group or any other group, take walks together.

- Join a birdwatching group or your Audubon Society chapter, so you can combine movement, nature, and community!

A NOTE ON COMMUNITY

By now you've got the big picture: our bodies benefit tremendously from movement. Want that picture to grow? Our bodies also require community. Humans are social animals by nature and for goldeners, a lack of social support can correlate with negative impacts on health (Donaldson and Watson 1996) and well-being (Singh and Misra 2009). Positive interaction with others can be important in reducing stress, increasing physical health, and reducing psychological issues such as depression and anxiety. And because it seems movement can do the same thing (Khazaee-Pool et al. 2015), why not double up and blend the two: community and more movement?

In addition to things like inviting a friend to come over and exercise with you, you can seek out group exercise classes or arrange to meet your friend for a walk. But again, it's not only about exercise; you can do this while moving more in your daily life as well.

Have you been choosing to drive through or use the ATM at

Joyce Says

I do movement work alone and find it enriching, and I also treasure the time I have moving with other people. In individual teaching I enjoy the one-to-one focus and problem solving together. And I simply love teaching group exercise classes. I work to incorporate humor when I'm teaching groups: it keeps me engaged with the class and with the process we are exploring together. Humor is the glue that binds us together with compassion and relief, hope and gratitude.

I welcome the opportunity to focus with someone in learning how their red flags of pain and trauma can be the doorways to their healing. While a group represents multiple points of view, bases of experience, different alignment point boundaries, and differing bases of resistance, I enjoy the challenge of helping the whole class relate to their work honestly and compassionately.

the bank for convenience? Parking and walking in not only increases your movement, it also offers the opportunity to interact with others as you wait in line (secretly practicing your standing alignment) and benefit from the smiles and interaction with those assisting you.

WALKING

- Increase your mileage.

- Increase the frequency of your walk.

- Stimulate your brain by changing your route.

- Add hills.

- Add various terrain.

- Add "vitamin Community."

 Joyce Says

Having lived in urban areas for the past fifty years, I have been challenged to give myself the wonderful benefits of daily walking in alignment. Here are some ideas from what I've learned over the last nine years of walking on sidewalks and streets with signals and stop signs, and crossing busy streets without those aids: Using the wait time at red signals to do either a Calf Stretch on a raised area of the sidewalk or a Pelvic List on each leg, checking my alignment as I walk, stand in line, or meet a friend and sit for lunch. I also seek out the unpaved portions of pedestrian walkways and choose to walk on them, benefiting from the uneven surfaces to massage the bottom of my feet, *(sidebar cont'd next page)*

(sidebar cont'd from previous page)

challenge my balance, and give relief to the unrelenting resistance of the concrete sidewalk surfaces.

My apartment building is located among dozens of similar buildings all connected with green areas, where mature sycamore, pine, and elm trees make a city forest. There's an adobe wall I can boost myself over on the way to the street, tree roots of all sizes and shapes that my feet love to feel, grass with soft and hard earth massaging my feet, and the challenge of hillocks gently and steeply ascending and descending. Gravel and rock surfaces give my feet a welcome challenge. Along the streets, some of the parkways are covered with mulch and/or gravel and pebbles, giving my body welcome relief from the hard sidewalks.

In some of the nearby large, multiple office building parks, there are spacious landscaped areas with grass and various sizes of boulders ready to be hopped on, and jumped to and from. There are lovely waterfalls integrated into the garden area to feast my eyes on. So I manage to get so much movement and nature time outdoors every day just navigating my neighborhood on foot to do my shopping, errands, teaching my classes, going to and from work, and meeting my friends for walks each week. I also get the benefit of the chemicals trees give off as my neighborhood is densely planted with a variety of trees, creating an urban forest.

(sidebar cont'd next page)

(sidebar cont'd from previous page)

In addition to enjoying the benefits of nature in an urban setting, I enjoy hiking and the beauty of nature walking outdoors at the nearby ocean, hills, and mountains. These areas offer a most glorious experience that is best consumed every day for me. The beauty of these areas is exhilarating and deeply nurturing. In such places I have free reign to find good climbing trees, hanging limbs and swinging limbs. There are roots in abundance, pebbles, rocks, boulders, and steep hills to climb for an hour or more, beautiful sandy beaches that challenge me to navigate wet, firm sand and dry, giving sand, and always the beckoning ocean for a swim and a visual bath in beauty.

Tweaking various alignment points as I walk, hike, and amble each day brings me healthy benefits: Do I need to tweak the outside edges of my feet to bring them straight? (Yes, most of the time.) Is my weight back in my heels? Am I pushing off with my butt muscles to move forward? Are my ribs centered? Is my head ramped? Do I have a plumb line from my ears to my hips?

These are some of the ways I have incorporated whole-body natural movement into my life. Good luck to you as you are motivated to find your healthy path.

WHOLE-BODY MOBILITY FLOW

You can always do exercises here and there, sprinkled throughout the day. A nice routine, however, can help focus your movement.

Equipment to have ready:

- chair

- rolled towel (or half foam roller)

- ball

- bolster (or pillows/blankets)

- hard flat-seated chair

(Please note detailed versions of the exercises can be found in the Exercise Glossary, which starts on page 191.)

Start standing and find your form: feet pelvis-width apart, weight back over heels, legs vertical, kneecaps relaxed, pelvis centered, ribs centered.

Look down and:

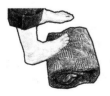

- Spread your toes

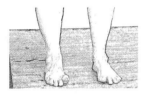

- Lift your big toes individually

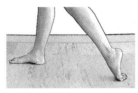

- Top of the Foot Stretch, repeat other side

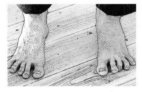

- Spread your toes again, lift and wiggle all your toes, lift your big toes individually

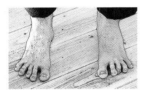

- Calf Stretch #1, repeat other side

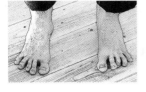

- Spread your toes again, lift and wiggle them, lift just the big toes

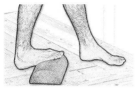

- Calf Stretch #2, repeat other side

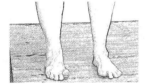

- Spread your toes, lift your big toes individually

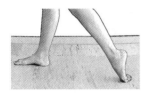

- Top of the Foot Stretch, repeat other side

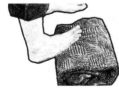

- Calf Stretch #1, repeat other side

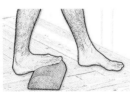

- Calf Stretch #2, repeat other side

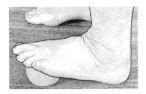

- Bottom of the Foot Stretch, repeat other side

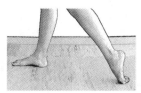 • Top of the Foot Stretch, repeat other side

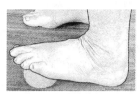 • Bottom of the Foot Stretch, repeat other side

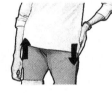 • The Pelvic List, repeat other side

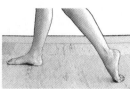 • Top of the Foot Stretch, repeat other side

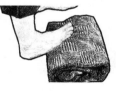 • Calf Stretch #1, repeat other side

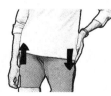 • The Pelvic List, repeat other side

 • Get up and down (from a chair or from the floor) three to four times

You can stop here, or, for more of a workout, stay down on your last "get down."

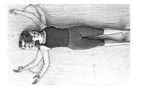

- Lie back on a bolster and do ten to twenty floor angels

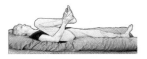

- Bring one knee in to reach your foot, repeat other side (if you're doing this on a chair, you can do this exercise on your bed at a later time)

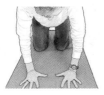

- Climb on to your hands and knees (use bolstering or padding as necessary), stretch your fingers and thumbs out, and rotate your elbows towards and away from each other to move your wrists and shoulders.

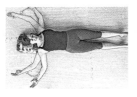

- Flip back over onto the bolster and do ten to twenty floor angels again

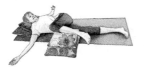

- Spinal Twist on bolster, repeat other side

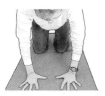

- Bring one knee in to reach your foot, repeat other side

- Flip back over on to your hands and knees to spread your fingers and rotate your elbows toward and away from each other

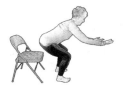

- Rise (pay attention to how you get up!) and sit in a chair

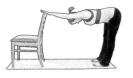

- Chair Squat four to five times

- Thoracic Stretch on wall or chair

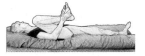

- Sit for Finger Stretches

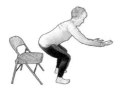 • Chair Squat four to five times (watch your shins and mind your form)

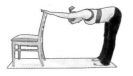 • Thoracic Stretch

 • Backing Up Twist, repeat other side

 • Elbow Touch

 • Finger Stretches

 • Elbow Touch, hold for five deep breaths

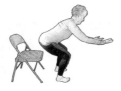

- Four to five Chair Squats

- On the last one, rise and walk to a door jamb and reach up to the top (or to the sides) and hold for four to five breaths, pulling down your ribs

- Stand on one leg and count to twenty, trying to not touch down (mind your form), and repeat other side.

Take a deep breath—you've moved your entire body!

EXERCISE GLOSSARY

Unless indicated otherwise, aim to do each of these exercises two to three times, for thirty seconds to a minute every time. **For any exercise requiring balance, stand near a wall or have a chair or something stable near by to hold on to.** Start every exercise by aligning yourself—feet straight and pelvis-width apart, kneecaps relaxed, pelvis and ribcage centered, and head ramped. If it's a sitting exercise, keep your knees over your ankles, feet straight, pelvis centered and ribs centered, and head ramped.

CHAPTER 1 EXERCISES

TOP OF THE FOOT STRETCH—SEATED

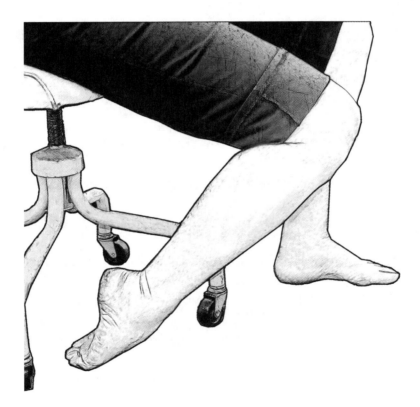

INSTRUCTIONS

- Sit near the front edge of a chair.

- Reach your right foot back to tuck under the toes.

- Keep your heel centered; don't let your ankles flop to the side.

- **Don't force the top of the foot to the floor in any way; allow your foot to lower as your muscles lengthen.**

- Repeat left side.

TOP OF THE FOOT STRETCH—STANDING

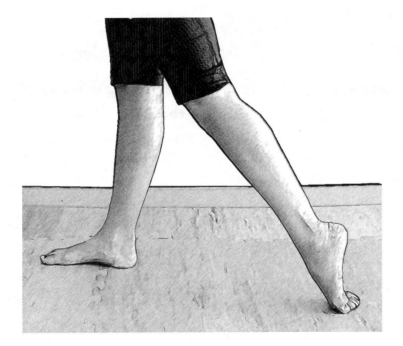

INSTRUCTIONS

- From standing, reach your right foot behind, tucking the toes under.

- Bring your chest and hips back so they stack over your non-stretching foot.

- To make the foot stretch less, shorten the distance you've reached the leg back.

- Repeat left side.

BOTTOM OF THE FOOT STRETCH

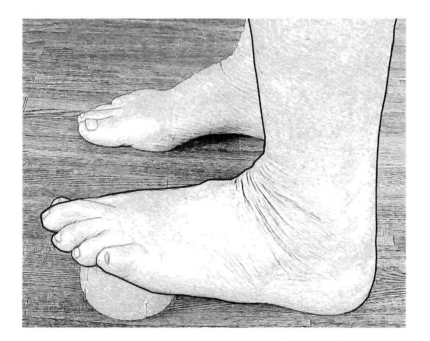

INSTRUCTIONS

- Sitting or standing, position a tennis or similarly sized squishy ball under the arch of one foot at a time.

- Slowly load your weight onto the ball (stay seated if necessary to reduce the load).

- Move your foot forward and back and side to side ("vacuuming" your foot) to gently articulate individual joints within the foot.

- Eventually, try different ball sizes and firmness.

PASSIVE TOE SPREADING

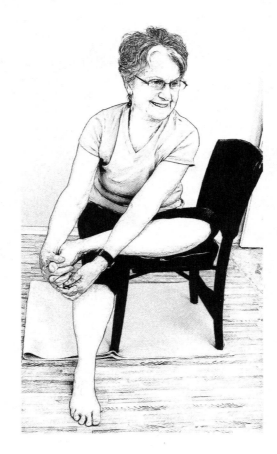

INSTRUCTIONS

- Sit with one ankle crossed over the opposite knee.

- With your hands, gently spread your toes apart, stretching the toes away from each other.

- To increase the stretch, push your fingers more deeply between the toes so that the webbing of your fingers and toes meet.

- To deepen even more, gently stretch your fingers apart, which will bring the toes with them.

- To lessen the stretch, do the reverse.

- Hold for up to a minute at a time.

- **If you're unsure about a limitation from a joint replacement or if your hips are too stiff to do this yet, see the options in the sidebar on page 37.**

ACTIVE TOE SPREADING

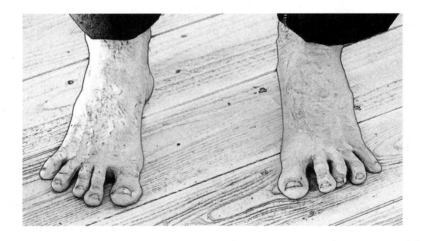

INSTRUCTIONS

- Stand with feet pelvis-width apart and pointing straight ahead, weight back in your heels.

- Spread your toes apart as far as you can, keeping all the toes flat on the ground.

- Repeat throughout the day (read: make sure your shoes aren't too tight to do this motion!).

TOE LIFTS

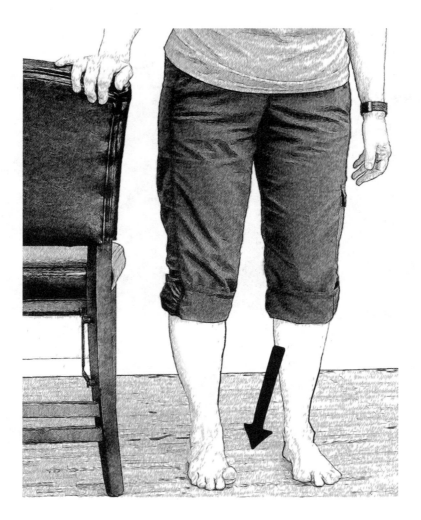

INSTRUCTIONS

- Lift your big toes while keeping the other eight toes on the ground.

- Then try lifting just the big toe on the left foot, and then the right.

- Work to lift each big toe straight upward, rather than letting it veer sideways (toward the pinkie toe).

- After you've mastered lifting your big toes, try lifting first them and then the second toe of each foot, making sure to keep the balls of your feet on the ground.

- Then lift the third, fourth, and fifth toes.

- Once all the toes are lifted, place them down one by one.

- Repeat, doing one foot at a time.

CHAPTER 2 EXERCISES

CALF STRETCH #1

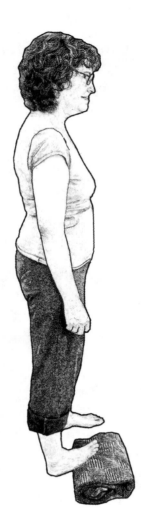

INSTRUCTIONS

- Place a thick folded and rolled towel (or a rolled yoga mat) on the floor in front of you.

- Step onto the towel with a bare or socked foot, placing the ball of the foot on the top of the towel.

- Adjust the foot so that it points straight forward, and slowly straighten your stretching leg.

- Keeping your body upright (try not to lean forward with your torso), step forward with the opposite foot.

- It's common to keep the non-stretching leg behind the towel at first. If you're leaning forward, finding you need to bend your knees, or losing your balance, shorten your stepping distance.

- More advanced: use a half foam roller instead of a rolled towel.

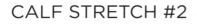

CALF STRETCH #2

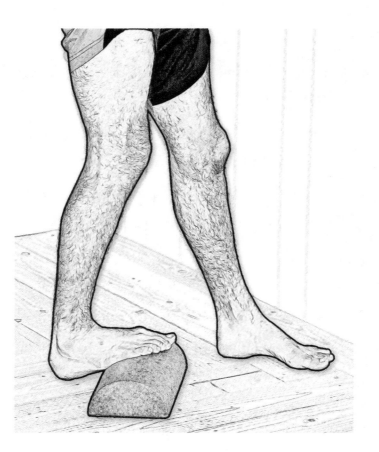

INSTRUCTIONS

- Beginning in the position of Calf Stretch #1, bend the knee of the foot on the rolled towel or half foam roller, pushing it slightly forward as you press that same heel toward the ground.

CHAPTER 3 EXERCISES

STANDING ON ONE LEG

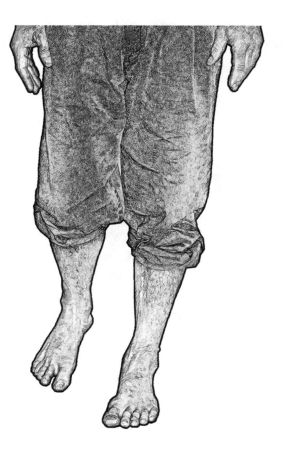

INSTRUCTIONS

- Holding lightly on to a wall or chair, try standing on one leg.

- Remove unnecessary tensions: relax your toes, back your hips up over your heels, straighten your knees without locking them (i.e., pulling up your kneecaps), drop your shoulders, and breathe in a relaxed way.

THE PELVIC LIST

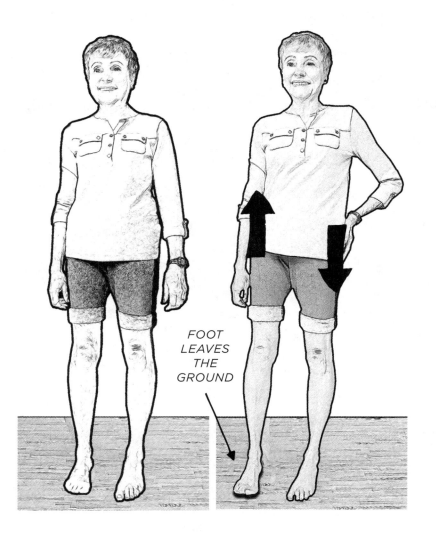

FOOT LEAVES THE GROUND

INSTRUCTIONS

- From aligned stance, place your right hand on your right hip and, using the muscles on the outside of the right hip, bring the right side of your pelvis down toward the floor (which will result in your left foot lifting away from the ground).

- If your left foot doesn't clear the ground, that's okay; keep practicing engaging these muscles until it does.

- Check to make sure you're not bending either knee, nor using the lower back of the floating side to lift the pelvis.

CHAPTER 5 EXERCISES

CHAIR SQUAT

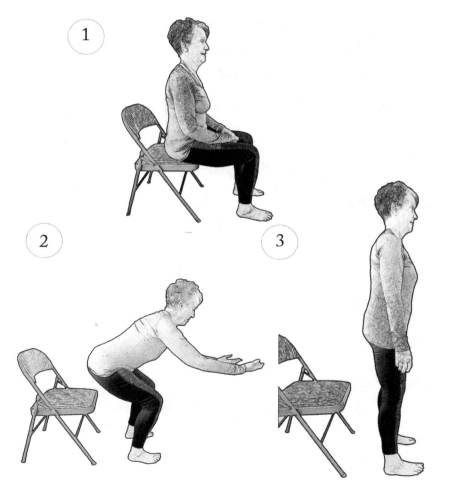

INSTRUCTIONS

- Sit on a flat, hard chair with pelvis untucked and ankles stacked directly below knees.

- Reaching your arms up and leaning your torso forward, shift your weight back into your heels as you stand up.

- Sit down slowly, weight still back in your heels.

- **If this is too difficult or causes any pain, stack towels or place a book or yoga block on the seat to give yourself a little lift.**

- As you get stronger, you can decrease the height of your bolster.

HOLD YOUR FEET

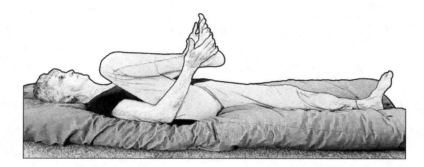

INSTRUCTIONS

- Lie on your back.

- Maintaining a relaxed breath, bring one knee toward your chest.

- Try to reach your foot with one and then both hands at once.

- Switch legs.

- Work up to being able to hold each foot in both hands in this position for one minute.

RAMP YOUR HEAD

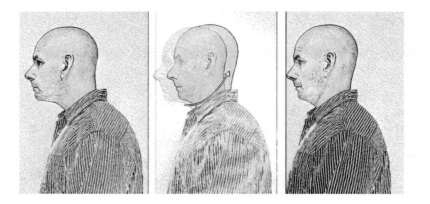

INSTRUCTIONS

- Without lifting it, slide your chin back until your ears align over your shoulders, lengthening the back of your neck.

FLOOR ANGELS

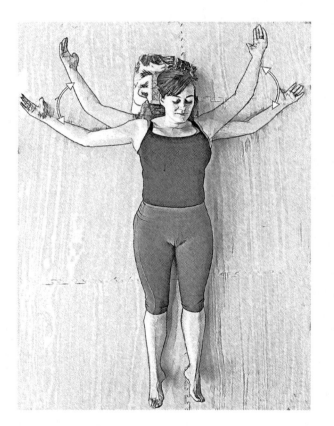

INSTRUCTIONS

- Begin by reclining on a bolster or stacked pillows so that the bottom of your ribcage can lower toward the floor.

- Straighten your legs.

- Reach your arms out to the sides, keeping your palms facing up and your elbows rotating up in the direction of the ceiling.

- Lower your arms and the backs of your hands toward the floor, keeping your elbows slightly bent.

- Once you've opened your arms as far as they can go, slowly move them up toward your head—like you're making snow angels.

- Try some however you can, and then try some only going as far as you can keeping your thumbs on the floor.

- Once you've done this for a while, try a few times monitoring your ribcage position—making sure that your ribs are staying down and not raising up as your arms move overhead.

THORACIC STRETCH

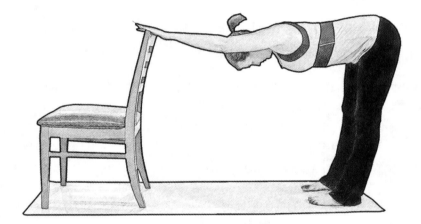

INSTRUCTIONS

- Stand facing a wall, countertop, or back of a chair (start higher and work your way down over time).

- Placing both hands on the wall (or whatever you've chosen), slowly back up until your arms are fully outstretched, lowering your chest through your arms.

- If you can, straighten your legs and shift your weight back toward your heels so you can easily wiggle your toes.

- Relax your head and neck.

DOORWAY REACH

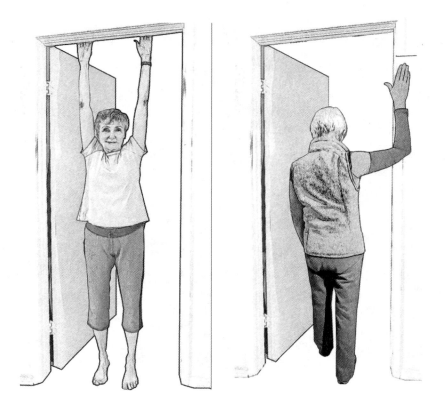

INSTRUCTIONS

- Reach your arms up until you can touch the wall above the doorway, and then lower your ribcage down as much as you can.

- If you can't do both arms at once, do one arm at a time, walking your fingers up the wall to the right of a doorway, as far as you can.

- Lowering your ribs will intensify the motion in your arms and shoulders.

- Repeat both sides.

- Check the position of your elbows. Do they always point outward? Try a few with your elbows pointing straight ahead and see how this movement changes the stretch in the arms, shoulders, and torso.

- Do this every time you go through a doorway, holding a few seconds each time.

STRENGTHEN THE MUSCLES BETWEEN YOUR RIBS

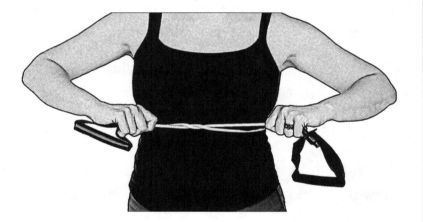

INSTRUCTIONS

- Seated or standing, tie an elastic band or pair of tights firmly around your ribcage, just beneath your chest muscles or breasts (at the height of a bra strap or heart-rate monitor).

- Center your ribs.

- Inhale deeply, expanding the ribcage into the band until you feel the resistance from the elastic pushing on your ribs. (If you don't feel it at the end of your inhale, re-tie the band a little more snugly and try it again.)

- Exhale, being aware of how your ribcage can pull away from the ring of elastic and closer to an imaginary vertical pole running up through the center of your body.

- Now instead of exhaling, try a slow cough in the same position, bringing the ribs inward.

- Repeat, using each exhale or cough to pull the ribs in and downward.

CHAPTER 6 EXERCISES

THE BACKING UP TWIST

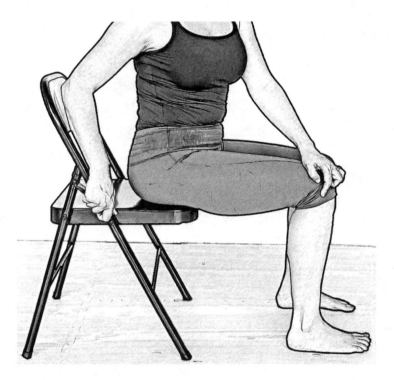

INSTRUCTIONS

- Seated, center your ribcage and pelvis.

- Without lifting your ribcage or tucking or untucking your pelvis, turn to the right without straining, and hold.

- Repeat other side.

BOLSTERED FLOOR TWIST

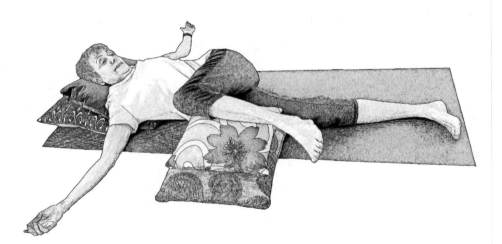

INSTRUCTIONS

- Lying on your back, bolster your upper body until your ribs are down.

- Scoot your pelvis an inch or two to the right, then bring the right knee up so that it stacks over your hip.

- Rotate your pelvis to lower that knee to the opposite side of your body, stopping as soon as your ribs start to lift away from the ground.

- **Twist only as far as you can without taking the ribs with you—no forcing it.**

- If you find that your pelvis barely moves and your knee is nowhere near the floor, **stack pillows so that the knee crossing over can rest on them.** This will reduce the load to the spine and keep these muscles from tensing unnecessarily.

- Repeat on the other side.

HANDS ON THE FLOOR (OR THE WALL)

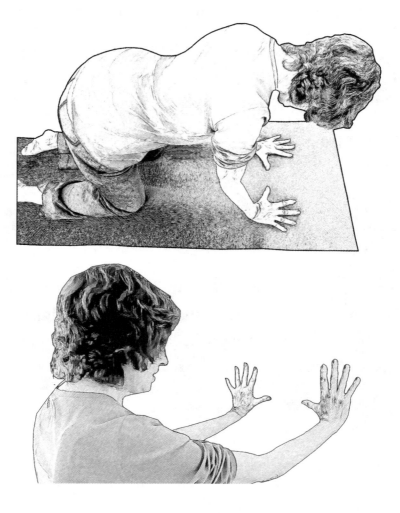

INSTRUCTIONS

- Get down on your hands and knees (**or, if that's not a feasible position for you right now, stand with your arms reaching forward to a wall**).

- Arrange your hands so that the middle finger on each hand is pointing straight forward (or straight up, if you're standing at a wall).

- Move your thumbs away from your fingers until they point directly toward each other, perpendicular to the middle fingers.

- Pull elbows inward with elbow pits facing forward, thumbs perpendicular and hands flat and relaxed (no finger joints bending, see "NO" picture below).

YES

NO *(FINGER JOINTS BENT)*

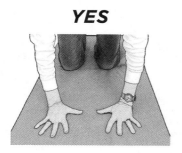
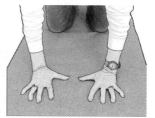

ELBOW TOUCH

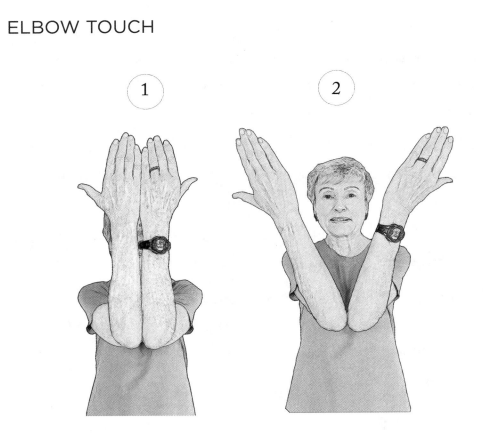

INSTRUCTIONS

- With your arms out in front of your body, elbows bent at 90° and palms facing you, bring your elbows together until they touch.

- Keeping the elbows together, move your wrists away from each other.

- Once you can do this with greater ease, lift your elbows (while keeping shoulders down).

FINGER STRETCHES

YES   _NO_

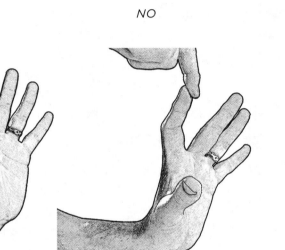

INSTRUCTIONS

- Place one hand out in front like you're signing STOP.

- Keeping that elbow bent and pointed to the ground, pull each finger back one at a time with your other hand until you feel a stretch.

- Pay close attention to the finger you are stretching to make sure none of its three joints are bending (see "no" picture).

APPENDIX: EXERCISE EQUIPMENT AND ADDITIONAL SOURCES OF INFORMATION

There are many places to obtain the equipment used in this book. Below are the places (or websites) from which I source my equipment for my home and studio. I've also included the recommended sizes for easiest ordering.

GENERAL EQUIPMENT

- **BOLSTER:** I recommend using a round bolster that is approximately 28 inches long with a 10 inch diameter. Find these sturdy cotton bolsters at YogaAccessories.com, your local yoga studio, or other online yoga supply companies.

- **HALF FOAM ROLLER:** I recommend using a 12x6x3 half foam roller (that's 12 inches long, 6 inches wide, and 3 inches tall). I order mine from foamerica.com. You can also find them on my website (nutritiousmovement.com/product/half-dome) as well as other exercise equipment stores.

- **SQUAT PLATFORM:** If you're interested in purchasing a squat platform for your toilet, I recommend the Squatty Potty. You can often find these at Costco, Bed Bath & Beyond as well as online at squattypotty.com.

- **YOGA BLOCK:** If you want to use a yoga block, I recommend using one that's 9x6x3 (9 inches long, 6 inches wide, and 3 inches tall). You can likely find these at your local yoga studio, sports equipment store, Target, or online at YogaAccessories.com.

EQUIPMENT AND INFORMATION FOR YOUR FEET

TOE SPACING DEVICES

- **FOAM TOE SEPARATORS**: Find inexpensive toe separators (typically used for pedicures) at any drugstore or pedicurist.

- **CORRECT TOES**: These toe spacers, which you can wear in shoes if your shoes are wide enough, are available at correcttoes.com.

- **FOOT ALIGNMENT SOCKS**: These toe-spacing socks are available at my-happyfeet.com.

TO MOVE THE BOTTOM OF YOUR FEET

- **TENNIS BALL**: Find them at any sporting good store.

- **YOGA TUNE UP™ BALLS**: These are great for the Bottom of the Foot Stretch as they're soft and designed for just this activity. You can find them, as well as video instructions on how to use them, at yogatuneup.com.

ADDITIONAL EXERCISES AND INFORMATION SPECIFIC TO SHOES AND FEET

FIND LISTS OF MINIMAL FOOTWEAR ON MY WEBSITE:

- Shoes: The List: nutritiousmovement.com/shoes-the-list

- Shoes: The Summer List: nutritiousmovement.com/shoes-the-summer-list

- Shoes: The Winter List: nutritiousmovement.com/shoes-the-winter-list

MY BOOKS ON THE MATTER:

- *Simple Steps to Foot Pain Relief: The New Science of Healthy Feet.* This is the more gentle introduction and focuses more on shoes.

- *Whole Body Barefoot: Transitioning Well to Minimal Footwear.* This book has many more exercises as well as more technical information on anatomy and biomechanics.

EQUIPMENT AND INFORMATION FOR YOUR PELVIC FLOOR

If you're currently experiencing pelvic floor issues, consider working with an alignment-aware physical therapist or physiotherapist with additional training in pelvic floor issues. You can request information on their training in pelvic floor matters to see if they're the best fit for you.

Exercises for pelvic alignment used by Shelah, Lora, Joyce, and Joan can be found in the following resources.

• In my exercise DVD *Nutritious Movement for a Healthy Pelvis* (find at nutritiousmovement.com).

• In my book *Diastasis Recti*, which, while dealing mainly with the core, also addresses pressures created through movement that constantly contribute to pelvic floor disorders.

When you've mastered the exercises here and feel like you're ready for more, you can find more advanced movements and habit changes in my book *Move Your DNA: Restore Your Health Through Natural Movement.* You can request any of these books at your local library or bookstore, or find them at any online retailer.

REFERENCES

American Geriatrics Society & A. Pomidor, Ed. 2016. *Clinician's Guide to Assessing and Counseling Older Drivers, 3rd Edition*. (Report No. DOT HS 812 228). Washington, DC: National Highway Traffic Safety Administration.

Balducci, S.; G. Iacobellis, L. Parisis, N. Di Biase, E. Calandriello, F. Leonetti, F. Fallucca. 2006. "Exercise training can modify the natural history of diabetic peripheral neuropathy." *Journal of Diabetes Complications* 20 (4): 216–23.

De Schryver, Anneke M., Yolande C. Keulemans, Harry P. Peters, Louis M. Akkermans, André J. Smout, Wouter R. De Vries, and Gerard P. Van Berge-Henegouwen. 2005. "Effects of Regular Physical Activity on Defecation Pattern in Middle-Aged Patients Complaining of Chronic Constipation." *Scandinavian Journal of Gastroenterology* 40(4): 422-429.

Donaldson, Jean M., and Robert Watson.1996. "Loneliness in Elderly People: An Important Area for Nursing Research." *Journal of Advanced Nursing 24(5):952–924.*

Fain, Elizabeth, and Cara Weatherford. 2016. "Comparative Study of Millennials' (Age 20–34 Years) Grip and Lateral Pinch with the Norms." *Journal Hand Therapy* 29(4): 483–488. doi: 10.1016/j.jht.2015.12.006.

Finlay, Jessica, Thea Franke, Heather McKay, Joanie Sims-Gould. 2015. "Therapeutic Landscapes and Wellbeing in Later Life: Impacts of Blue and Green Spaces for Older Adults." *Health & Place* 34: 97–106.

Friedman, Susan M., Beatriz Munoz, Sheila K. West, Gary S. Rubin, Linda Fried. 2002. "Falls and Fear of Falling: Which Comes First? A Longitudinal Prediction Model Suggests Strategies for Primary and Secondary Prevention." *Journal of the American Geriatrics Society* 50(8): 1329–1335.

Greenman, R., L. Khaodhiar, C. Lima, T. Dinh, J. Giurini, A. Veves. 2005. "Foot Small Muscle Atrophy Is Present Before the Detection of Clinical Neuropathy." *Diabetes Care* 28(6): 1425–1430.

Hausdorff, Jeffrey M., Becca R. Levy, Jeanne Y. Wei. 1999. "The Power of Ageism on Physical Function of Older Persons: Reversibility of Age-Related Gait Changes." *Journal of the American Geriatrics Society* 47(11): 1346–1349.

Herman, T., N. Giladi, T. Gurevick, and J. M. Hausdorff. 2005. "Gait Instability and Fractal Dynamics of Older Adults with a 'Cautious' Gait: Why Do Certain Adults Walk Fearfully?" *Gait and Posture* 21(2): 178–185.

Khazaee-Pool, M., R. Sadeghi, F. Majlessi, and A. Rahimi Foroushani. 2015. "Effects of Physical Exercise Programme on Happiness Among Older People." *Journal of Psychiatric and Mental Health Nursing* 22: 47–57.

Lach, H. W. 2005. "Incidence and Risk Factors for Developing Fear of Falling in Older Adults. *Public Health Nursing*, 22 (1): 45–52.

Mayo Clinic. 2016. "Poor Diet and Lack of Exercise Accelerate the Onset of Age-Related Conditions in Mice." ScienceDaily.

NIH Senior Health. n.d. "Falls and Older Adults: Causes and Risk Factors." <nihseniorhealth.gov/falls/causesandriskfactors/01.html>

Park, B. J., Y. Tsunetsugu, T. Kasetani, T. Kagawa, and Y. Miyazaki. 2009. "The Physiological Effects Of Shinrin-Yoku (Taking In the Forest Atmosphere or Forest Bathing): Evidence From Field Experiments in 24 Forests Across Japan." *Environmental Health and Preventive Medicine* 15(1): 18-26. doi:10.1007/s12199-009-0086-9.

Shull, Pete B., Rebecca Shultz, Amy Silder, Jason L. Dragoo, Thor F. Besier, Mark R. Cutkosky, Scott L. Delp. 2013. "Toe-In Gait Reduces the First Peak Knee Adduction Moment in Patients With Medial Compartment Knee Osteoarthritis." *Journal of Biomechanics* 46(1): 122–128.

Sherrington, C., and H. B. Menz. 2003. "An Evaluation of Footwear Worn At the Time of Fall-Related Hip Fracture." *Age and Ageing* 32(3): 310-4.

Singh, Archana, and Nishi Misra. 2009. "Loneliness, Depression and Sociability in Old Age." *Industrial Psychiatry Journal* 18.1: 51–55. PMC. Web. 10 Dec. 2016.

Smith, J. Carson et al. 2014. "Physical Activity Reduces Hippocampal Atrophy in Elders at Genetic Risk for Alzheimer's Disease." *Frontiers in Aging Neuroscience* 6: 61.

Strickler, Jeff. 2015. "95-year-old shares tricks of safe falling." *Star Tribune*, March 2. <startribune.com/95-year-old-shares-tricks-of-safe-falling/294726671/>

University of Minnesota. 2015. "Everyday Access to Nature Improves Quality of Life in Older Adults." [press release]. <twin-cities.umn.edu/news-events/everyday-access-nature-improves-quality-life-older-adults>

Zheng, Selin J., N. Orsini, Lindblad B. Ejdervik, and A. Wolk. 2015. "Long-Term Physical Activity and Risk of Age-Related Cataract: A Population-Based Prospective Study of Male and Female Cohorts." *Ophthalmology* 122 (2): 274–80.

INDEX

H

I

J

K

L

M

Mayo Clinic, 162

mindfulness, 18, 19, 31, 99, 112, 135

N

national parks, 10, 25

neuropathy, *see* foot ailments

neutral knee-pits, 76-78

NIH, 49, 51

O

obstacles, 100-103

orthotics, 23-25

osteoarthritis/osteoporosis, 22, 59, 162

P

pain
 - versus new sensations, 18
 - *see also* chronic pain

pelvic floor/pelvic floor disorders, 2, 9-10, 79, 91, 135, 241-242

Pelvic List, 83, 85-87, 105, 176, 180, 186, 210-211

pelvis tucking, *see* tucking of the pelvis

Pillow Train, 99, 102-103

prolapse of pelvic organs, *see* pelvic floor/pelvic floor disorders

prostate issues, *see* pelvic floor/pelvic floor disorders

purposeful walking, 100

R

Rapid-Pace Walking Test, 151

reaching your toes, 132, 172-173, 187, 188

textured ground, *see* vitamin texture

Thoracic Stretch, 123, 188, 189, 220-221

toe gripping/clenching, 26, 47, 80, 104-105

Toe Lifts, 42-43, 48, 153, 184-185, 202-203

Toe Spreading, 35-41, 153

toileting, 133-134, 174, 238

Top of the Foot Stretch, 29-30, 43, 155, 184, 185, 186, 192-195

tucking of the pelvis, 79, 91, 141, 213, 227

U

urinating, *see* toileting

V

vitamin Community, 96-97, 180

vitamin Nature, 97-99

vitamin Texture, 99

W

walking

 - buddy/group, 97, 177

 - creating more challenge, 94-96

 - mechanics of, 90-94

 - *see also* gait

weight back on your heels, 25, 27-28, 78-80, 90, 110, 117, 169, 176, 182, 184

Whole Body Barefoot, 21, 240

workstation, *see* computer

ACKNOWLEDGMENTS

Thanks to Joan Virginia Allen, whose bold vision and leadership brought our group into being; and to Shelah and Lora, my sister septuagenarians, for their courage and honesty. The four of us inspired each other as we met monthly to record how our lives were transformed so others experiencing physical limitations would know there is another choice available—one of healing the cause. What a welcome and radical choice in our culture dominated by symptom control.

—J. F.

Aging dynamically has been and is motivated by special people in my life, including, but not limited to, my mom and dad, Virginia and Ted, who modeled *dynamic aging*; my younger brother and sister, Jerry and Linda, and their spouses, Marilyn and Ken; my beautiful children, Camela, Craig, Wendy, and Jasmine; my eight awesome grandchildren, Tyler, Dashiel, Zoe, Nicholas, Cameron, Graham, Connor, and Liam; and my three savvy, sassy septuagenarian "sisters," Joyce, Shelah, and Lora, with whom I lovingly share our individual and unique experiences of *dynamic aging*.

—J. V. A.

Thanks to John Eder Photography, who brought us to life. And to Joanne Krantz, whose request for written material to assist her in both her long-distance mothers' balance assaults prompted us to create this book.

—L. W.

Thank you to my late husband, Estel, the best partner ever. I miss you! Also to my septuagenarian sisters, Joan, Joyce and Lora, and my chosen sisters, Pam, Tessa, and Nancy, who make my life so much richer. The sisters I always wanted! And thanks to my dear children, Celeste, Tao, Evan and Brad. Your kindness, love and patience are exemplary. So proud of each of you.

—S. W.

ABOUT THE AUTHORS

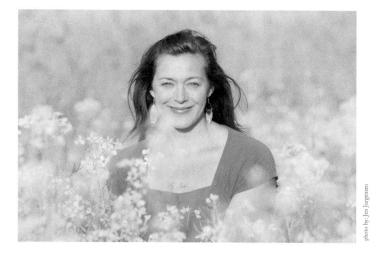

photo by: Jen Jurgensen

Part biomechanist, part science communicator, and full-time mover, Katy Bowman has educated hundreds of thousands of people on the role movement plays in the body and in the world. Blending a scientific approach with straight talk about sensible, whole-life movement solutions, her website and award-winning podcast, *Katy Says*, reach hundreds of thousands of people every month, and thousands have taken her live classes.

Her books, the bestselling *Move Your DNA*, *Movement Matters*, *Simple Steps to Foot Pain Relief*, *Diastasis Recti*, *Don't Just Sit There*, *Whole Body Barefoot*, *Alignment Matters*, and *Every Woman's Guide to Foot Pain Relief*, have been critically acclaimed and translated worldwide.

Passionate about human movement outside of exercise, Katy volunteers her time to support the larger reintegration of movement into human lives by providing movement courses across widely varying demographics and working with non-profits promoting nature education. She also directs and teaches at the Nutritious Movement™ Center Northwest in Washington state, travels the globe to teach Nutritious Movement courses in person, and spends as much time outside as possible with her husband and children.

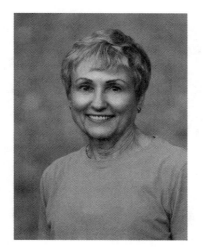

In her seventy-ninth year, Joan Virginia Allen is experiencing dynamic aging in her teaching, hiking, tree climbing and hanging, and sharing her vitality and *joie de vivre* with her husband, children, grandchildren, siblings, and friends. Joan is a retired attorney, actress, author, and speaker who lives in Ojai, California.

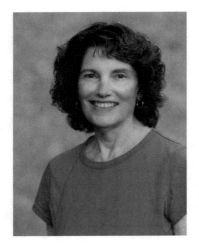

Shelah Wilgus is a graphic designer, fiber artist, and aspiring photographer who's trying to save the planet by promoting a plant-based lifestyle and teaching vegan cooking classes. She loves working with older people (she is one), digitally restoring old photographs, exploring the world on her two feet, and doing the Calf Stretch. She lives in Ventura, California.

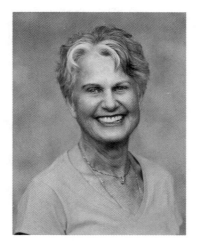

Joyce Faber is a passionate third-generation teacher, mother, stepmother, grandmother, and great-grandmother. Her lifelong love of teaching has evolved from avidly seeking/teaching wisdom and health to living with mobility into her eighties practicing whole-body movement. She enjoys passing on what she's learned from Katy Bowman, teaching senior classes, and hiking in the outdoors with friends and family. She lives in Ventura, California.

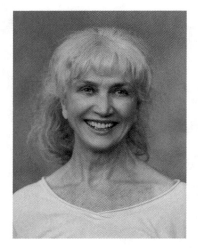

Lora Woods is beginning her seventy-sixth year on earth, now older than any known progenitor. She works hard to do right by the earth, while the stars in her personal universe are Randy, Amanda and Thomas Sherren. Lora lives in Ojai, California, where everything is accessible by foot and hiking is awesome.